Towards Newborn Survival

"This book successfully addressed the evidence gap in barriers to newborn survival in Bihar using scientific inquiry and sound analytical techniques. I am confident that such scientific exploration of grass root experiences will immensely benefit researchers, practitioners and would contribute towards evidence-based policy making especially in resource poor settings."

—Prof. K.S. James, Director, *IIPS, Mumbai*

"This book conveys an understanding of new-born care in a regional perspective towards identifying strategies and policies for betterment in an underdeveloped setting."

—Prof. U.S. Mishra, *IIPS, Mumbai*

Sandhya R. Mahapatro

Towards Newborn Survival

Challenges and Priorities

palgrave
macmillan

Sandhya R. Mahapatro
A.N.Sinha Institute of Social Studies
Patna, India

ISBN 978-981-19-3416-2 ISBN 978-981-19-3417-9 (eBook)
https://doi.org/10.1007/978-981-19-3417-9

This Palgrave Macmillan imprint is published by the registered company Springer Nature Singapore Pte Ltd.
The registered company address is: 152 Beach Road, #21-01/04 Gateway East, Singapore 189721, Singapore

Contents

List of Figures

List of Tables

CHAPTER 1

Newborn Health: An Introduction

Background

The neonatal period, spanning the first 28 days of life after birth, is the most crucial period of child health as it carries the highest risk of mortality. Estimates show the mortality risk of a neonate is 30-fold higher than that of an under-five child (Sankar et al. 2016). Globally, newborn deaths account for almost half (47 per cent) of under-five deaths (Suzuki and Kashiwase 2020). The UN IGME report (2017) on 'Levels and Trends in Child Mortality' finds although under-five death has decreased, the proportion of under-five death in the neonatal period increased from 41 per cent in 2000 to 46 per cent in 2016. An acceleration in the reduction of under-five deaths for achieving the SDG targets calls for a focus on newborn survival. Pregnancy and childbirth are events of great happiness for families. Higher newborn deaths exert pressure on families to produce more children, which negatively impacts mother's health and in turn household economy and well-being. A healthy start for every newborn is vital for a country's growth and development, as it is related to its demography, human capital, and poverty reduction. Reduction in neonatal deaths is crucial for the overall well-being and, as such, is being increasingly recognised as a public health priority. Both MDGs and SDGs emphasise on good health for mothers and children for a healthy life and well-being at all ages. The SDG target for neonatal mortality rate (NMR) is to reduce it to 12 per 1000 live births by 2030.

S. R. Mahapatro, *Towards Newborn Survival*,
https://doi.org/10.1007/978-981-19-3417-9_1

Newborn survival is a major challenge for low- and middle-income countries (Tinker et al. 2005). While Latin America, the Caribbean, and Central/Eastern Europe have made substantial progress in bringing neonatal mortality down, the rate of neonatal deaths continues to be high in sub-Saharan Africa and South Asian countries (UNICEF 2014). Newborn deaths in low-income countries (LIC) are almost nine times higher than in high-income settings (Hug et al. 2019) and also account 99 per cent of total neonatal death (Lawn et al. 2005). Estimates show most newborn deaths occurred in Southern Asia (39 per cent) and sub-Saharan Africa (38 per cent), with India, Pakistan, Nigeria, the Democratic Republic of the Congo, and Ethiopia accounting for half of these deaths (UN IGME 2017). The average annual rate of decline in neonatal mortality was found to be 2.6 per cent between 1990 and 2018, a smaller decrease compared to under-five mortality rate (3.6 per cent) (WHO 2020).

India ranks 12th among 52 lower- and middle-income nations on NMR (UNICEF 2018) and the third highest (22.7 per cent) among the South Asian countries after Pakistan and Afghanistan (UN IGME 2019). In recent years, the country has recorded a higher NMR (28 vs. 18 per 1000 live births) than the global average and accounted for over a quarter of the world's 2.6 million neonatal deaths (Kapoor et al. 2020). The burden of neonatal deaths is nearly three-fourth (71 per cent) of total infant deaths and the decline is relatively slower than infant and under-five mortality. It appears that the country has a long way to go to achieve the SDG goal pertaining to NMR. An acceleration in its pace of decline is deemed to be vital for progress towards SDG 3.2 as also the India Newborn Action Plan of reducing NMR to a single digit by 2030. Bending the NMR trend will require a laser-sharp focus on addressing the barriers that affect newborn survival in the regions that recorded more deaths among neonates.

Demographically, India is the second most populous country in the world and population explosion is a major concern for development. The neo-classical theorist, like Malthus[1], Ehrlich[2] argued that growing population exerts an accelerated strain on the natural world; hence, population control through fertility declines and child survival is important. The role

[1] Malthus in his book *An Essay on Principles of Population* warned that theoretically the human population grows exponentially, while the resources tend to grow arithmetically, resulting in poverty, misery, and poor health.

[2] Ehrlich in his book *The Population Bomb* advocated for immediate attention to be paid to population control.

of demographic parameters of fertility and mortality in influencing population size, health, and development has its historical significance and is highlighted in the theory of demographic transition—the demographic shift from high to low levels of fertility and mortality. In traditional societies, mortality crisis surfaced with famine, and natural calamities appeared as the barriers to population control. The classical theorists of demographic transition postulate that infant and child mortality decline is a prerequisite for lower fertility rates. Over the course of demographic transition, fertility decline was emphasised as an immediate measure of population control; however, this might be as a response of couples to the improvement in survival chances of offspring (Tymicki 2009). If the fertility goal of a couple could not accomplish due to mortality risk, they may go for more children. To change the reproductive trends in a high fertility context, infant and child survival is, therefore, of particular importance. While, supporting the hypothesis of child survival, studies have shown that a decline in child mortality, in tandem with the socioeconomic transition, is a precondition for fertility transition (Cleland 2001; Ranganathan et al. 2015). India has undergone rapid demographic changes in recent decades, with considerable heterogeneity between the states. While the southern states of Kerala and Tamil Nadu are demographically advantaged and reached replacement level of fertility, in the northern states of Bihar and Uttar Pradesh, such transition is still underway. Attaining replacement level of fertility thus calls for an accelerated reduction in neonatal and infant mortality in such states.

The significance of health for the nation's development has been realised since the early days of independence. During the British regime, India had no official policy on population health. The Bhore committee report (1946), for the first time, emphasised incorporating public health in the developmental strategies and recommended investing in the public health infrastructure for improving health outcomes. The recommendations of the committee became a part of India's developmental strategies, beginning with the implementation of the five-year plans in 1951. While the five-year plans did focus on various aspects of health, a higher priority was accorded to family planning measures for birth control. This strongly influenced the political regime until the Congress Party was routed out of power in 1977. In 1979, the Planning Commission set up a working group to formulate long-term plans for population policy; it was then that the focus shifted from crude birth rate (CBR) to net reproduction rate (NRR) (Srinivasan 2017). While taking the historical as well as the recent experience into account, the working group realised that lower birth rates had never been achieved without a reduction in the death rate, specifically in infants. Maternal and child healthcare was, thus, prioritised for the first time in the seventh five-year plan (1985–1990). The programmes implemented under this plan were integrated into the Child Survival and Safe Motherhood programme in the eighth five-year plan (1992–1997).

Maternal and child health agenda was reiterated in the International Conference on Population and Development (ICPD) held in Cairo (1994). It was a paradigm shift in the field of reproductive health with a wider focus from family planning to reproductive rights, gender equity, and empowerment. In ICPD it was recommended that strategies and interventions under population policies should not be formulated solely considering the fertility concern; rather they should be engendered by prioritising the reproductive health and rights of women. The Indian government, being a signatory, introduced the Reproductive Health Approach in 1997. Following that, the National Population Policy (NPP), 2000 and the National Health Policy (NHP), 2002 were implemented in the country; all efforts had been geared to reduce maternal and infant mortality. In 2005, the National Rural Health Mission (NRHM) was launched as a flagship programme by the then-Honourable Prime Minister, Dr Manmohan Singh, under the United Progressive Alliance (UPA) government. Since then, the health sector has been on a reform path in providing universal healthcare to all. With massive investments in infrastructure and the adoption of a more synergistic approach to understanding the determinants of health, the health system has significantly influenced the mother and child health indicators in a positive manner.

The evolution of healthcare reforms in India, however, has not resulted in sufficient attention being paid to neonatal mortality. High NMR has remained a neglected problem in various policy and planning documents despite the neonatal period being a critical phase of infant survival. One of the reasons for such neglect could be the inequality in the NMR across the states with a demographically varied structure. States experiencing the late phase of demographic transition report a lower NMR than those that are in the early phase. For instance, while NMR is 5 per 1000 live births in Kerala, it is almost 4 to 5 times higher in the EAG states. In 2014, the India Newborn Action Plan was implemented to reduce preventable neonatal deaths. Despite an overall improvement in under-five mortality, a stagnancy in neonatal mortality, specifically in the socioeconomically backward states, continues to be observed. A study by Bora and Saikia (2018) finds nearly half of the districts in India located mainly in poorer states are unlikely to achieve the SDG targets in NMR. Given the complexity of environment, a woman experiences and lives in that, exploring causal forces—both societal and structural—that affect newborn survival is critical for achieving the SDG targets.

Neonatal mortality assumes special significance in the demographic research as the intensity of events (deaths) and causes of death (combined exogenous and endogenous determinants) differ in many aspects from infant and child mortality. The survival of a newborn is not only conditioned by biological or medical factors, but also by a multitude of socioeconomic, cultural, and systemic ones. Access to and utilisation of quality healthcare in continuum from the inception of pregnancy to the first four weeks after birth critically influences the mortality risk of neonates. The theoretical approaches to healthcare utilisation underline the significance of social determinants with respect to healthcare use. The health belief model developed in the 1950s (Hochbaum et al. 1952) attempted to link health behaviours with certain belief patterns. It emphasised that the use of healthcare depends on perceived susceptibility to illness, perceived severity of contracting an illness and its consequences, perceived benefits of action, perceived barriers to actions, and cues to action. This model deals only with the factors affecting the healthcare behaviour of individuals of all age groups. Biological as well as environmental conditions, or the service delivery mechanisms, however, also wrought the use of healthcare. The analytical framework of child survival proposed by Mosley and Chen underscores the significance of the socioeconomic, medical, and environmental determinants and their interaction in explaining child survival. As per the framework, the mechanisms underlying the functioning of the socioeconomic determinants that result in differential mortality patterns remain unexplained in the literature. The above two models offer only a partial understanding of the significance of behavioural factors—culture or norms in the local context—and institutional factors and their intricate association with socioeconomic conditions in deciding child health. Besides, neither of them focuses exclusively on newborn health, which is different from child health in many ways.

Research studies though documented prevalence and estimation of NMR (Arokiasamy and Gautam 2008; Neogi et al. 2015) or examined the correlates of neonatal mortality, less emphasis was given to exploring the contextual adversities that jeopardise newborn health. In some social environments, the decision to seek care is influenced by beliefs, cultural practices, and perceived barriers to care (Loke et al. 2015) and is not confined to health system performances. The supply of healthcare services and more specifically improved quality of care undoubtedly has a great impact on the use of newborn care (Fadel et al. 2015). Thus, newborn health and chances of survival should be understood taking into account both the demand- and supply-side aspects, including socioeconomic, maternal, cultural, biomedical, and institutional factors. While there is a growing recognition that social and structural barriers influence newborn survival, the pathways that jeopardise newborn health are incompletely understood. This calls for a more detailed analysis so as to address the impediments to newborn health.

India, the most populous country of South Asia, comprises socioeconomically and demographically advantaged and disadvantaged states. A blanket approach to understand the attributes influencing NMR may not give a clear picture in a diverse socioeconomic context. Large-scale survey-based enquiries are unable to cover the realities associated with newborn care in specific socio-cultural contexts. This underscores the importance of investigating the mechanisms that influence newborn health at the local level. Studies examining the intricate interplay between socioeconomic vulnerability and health system challenges with regard to newborn health are scarce in demographic literature. The micro-level enquiry presented in this book offers an opportunity for exploration of the contextual barriers in greater detail.

The Significance of the Study Area: Bihar

A considerable progress in neonatal survival is needed for India to achieve the SDG 3.2 of reducing the NMR to 12 per 1000 live births. This is particularly challenging for the state of Bihar for two specific reasons. One, it has the highest Total Fertility Rate of 3.0 (National Family Health Survey-5) among all the states of India and lags in the demographic transition. Two, it is far away from achieving the SDG targets on account of the conditions required to achieve the neonatal outcomes. These challenges are exacerbated by the high levels of illiteracy, poverty, inequalities, and the rigid social norms that prevail in the state. NMR has remained mostly stagnant in Bihar over time; however, it declined by 10 per cent between 2017 and 2018 from 28 to 25 per 1000 live births, but was higher than the national average of 23 per 1000 live births (SRS 2018).

In the last few years, many interventions have been implemented and the state has been continuously allocating a substantial share of its budget[3] towards refurbishing the health system by strengthening the infrastructure, improving the delivery of quality services, and increasing the access to services. Despite these significant gains, prevention and reduction of neonatal mortality is still a challenge for the health system. To meet the targets enshrined in the SDG, neonatal mortality needs to decline by more than half in the state. Reduction in NMR, therefore, deserves special attention, and an exploration of the impediments to newborn survival is critical in this direction. The micro analysis presented in this book allows for an exploration of the local attributes such as beliefs, practices, and cultural norms, alongside the health system barriers in influencing newborn survival.

The present study uses the Mosley and Chen (1984) framework, with modifications based on the literature. The framework proposed here (Fig. 1.1) states that socioeconomic and demographic factors influence the health-seeking behaviour directly or through an interaction with the supply-side measures to determine newborn survival. Figure 1.1 intends to show the pathways of newborn survival through the utilisation of services and care practices with three embedded constructs: (1) Socio-demographic factors that focus on household and maternal attributes; (2) institutional factors that include providers' attributes such as quality of delivery and effectiveness of programmes and policies; and (3) health beliefs—that include perceived benefits, perceived severity of illness, and perceived barriers—that are shaped by the local contextual factors. It can be assumed that the beliefs, misconceptions, and practices prevailing in the community that influence the decisions on healthcare are also shaped by education, wealth status, and caste differences. At the same time, the quality of care received in institutions influences the perception about seeking further care. The interaction of these pathways ultimately affects women's care-seeking behaviour, from the onset of pregnancy to the neonatal period, which are both crucial to newborn health.

[3]The JDU-led government, within a span of 15 years, has increased the health department's budget to 10,000 crore in 2020 from 278 crore in 2005. (https://www.deccanherald.com/national/east-and-northeast/bihar-health-budget-increased-to-rs-10000-cr-in-15-years-minister-883561.html). For the year 2020–2021, the state has allocated 5.2 per cent of the total budget to health, which is slightly lower than the state average of 5.3 per cent.

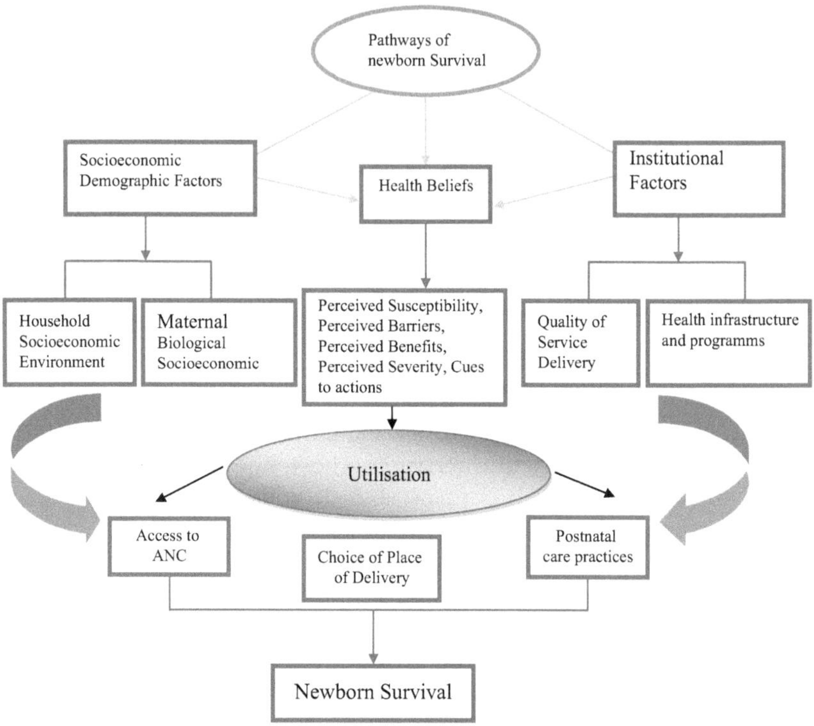

Fig. 1.1 Conceptual framework of pathways of newborn survival

A closer investigation into various aspects of neonatal health in the continuum will provide insights into the barriers that affect utilisation of newborn services and cause neonatal deaths in the state. From policy perspective, designing strategic interventions for newborn survival, an improved understanding of the barriers that obstruct utilisation of newborn health services is significant. It is envisaged that a clear inspection of such dynamics is key to building a responsive healthcare system tailored to the needs of mothers and children and to eventually improving health outcomes in Bihar.

Objectives

The primary focus of the book is to unfold the structural and societal barriers that cause poor health outcomes of newborns. Although health system factors are important to ensure improved neonatal health outcome, it is imperative to understand the socio-cultural context of women that impacted health-seeking behaviour. The broader question posed is: Are the barriers to newborn health primarily related to societal causes (demand side) or are they health sector constraints (supply), or is there an intersection of both demand- and supply-side barriers? The specific questions that will be explored in this context are: What are the local contextual adversities that shape newborn service utilisation? Do the underprivileged grapple with an elevated risk of neonatal mortality? Are the health system resources adequate and equitable to address the barriers to newborn health services? What are the challenges that affect successful programme delivery? This will provide what factors are placing mother and newborn at health risk.

The specific objectives are:

- Firstly, to understand the social determinants of NMR for India and in the Empowered Action Group states. Here we identify the factors affecting newborn health and the variations across the regions within India.
- Secondly, to systematically explore the interplay of socio-cultural and system-level barriers that jeopardise newborn health. This objective will answer the research question raised about the contextual barriers to newborn health and examine how far socioeconomic inequities and health system adversities affect access to service utilisation.
- Lastly, to analyse the role of healthcare interventions in changing traditional care practices and increasing service utilisation, and to understand implementation challenges. This will answer the question on the barriers to the uptake of various services, the impact of programmes on newborn health, and the challenges to the effective implementation of programmes.

Data and Method

The analyses in this book relied mostly on data collected from the field survey. Data drawn from secondary sources such as the Sample Registration System (SRS) and the National Family Health Survey (NFHS), 2015 were also utilised to set the background of the study. The SRS has been providing estimates of fertility and mortality on a regular basis since 1970. The NFHS is the Demographic and Health Survey (DHS) of India that collects detailed information on maternal and child healthcare indicators. Four rounds of the NFHS have been carried out in India so far. The latest round, NFHS-5, was in 2019–2020; however, it provides details about a few states only as the data collection process is still underway. A comparable assessment of the health situation across the states could be made only through large-scale survey-based enquiries like NFHS. To make a situational assessment of the health infrastructure available, secondary sources of data from the Health Management Information System (HMIS) were used. These secondary data sources, however, would not have been able to capture the micro-level realities that influence maternal and newborn health. To explore the access barriers to newborn survival and the implementation challenges of interventions, data collected from the primary survey was analysed.

Bivariate and multivariate analyses were performed to understand the newborn health situation. Descriptive statistics, including rates, ratio, correlation, and chi-square tests, were used to understand the association of various socioeconomic and programmatic indicators with neonatal mortality. While chi-square tests were used to establish the statistical significance of the association, Principal Component Analysis (PCA) was used to compute the autonomy index of women and the wealth index of the household. Multivariate analysis has also been performed to explore the linkages of socioeconomic realities with NMR.

Criteria for Selection of Study Area

Following the multistage stratified random sampling technique, eight districts of Bihar were selected based on the level of institutional delivery as per NFHS-4 and classified into the following ranges: Less than 60, 60–69, 70–79, and 80 and above, and from each category, two sample districts were further selected. The districts of Jehanabad and Rohtas had a high prevalence of institutional delivery, whereas Madhubani and Kishanganj recorded the lowest. The Census of India 2011 was used as the sampling frame for the study. The Primary Sampling Units (PSUs) were census villages in the case of rural areas, and wards in the case of urban areas. Irrespective of the rural-urban population ratio, the number of rural and urban PSUs was fixed. In the first stage, all the villages and wards of a district were stratified into four strata based on the percentage of the scheduled caste population as less than 25, 26–50, 51–75, and 75 and above. Using the Probability Proportional to Population Size (PPS) technique, the number of PSUs for each of the stratum was determined; the PSUs were then selected using systematic sampling. In total, 16 PSUs were selected from each of the 8 districts.

In the second stage, circular systematic sampling was adopted for selecting the households. The mapping and listing of the households, which served as the sampling frame for the survey, was carried out in each PSU following the preparation of the location and layout maps for village segmentation. Larger villages, with more than 200 households, were segmented into one or more segments, and each segment covering a minimum of 200 households was selected for the listing and mapping. As per the rural-urban population ratio, the PSUs were divided into 115 rural and 13 urban PSUs. The study, therefore, covered a total of 128 sample PSUs, 16 PSUs from each district represented by 20 households and total sample comprised 2384 households. The size of the sample was fixed to get reliable estimates of neonatal mortality at the state and district levels at a reasonable cost. The households selected for the survey had at least one eligible woman in the age group 15–49 years who had given birth during one year preceding the survey date. The study sample was chosen to be representative of the state in explaining the maternal and newborn health situation.

Along with the household, 64 facilities and 109 communities were also surveyed. The selection of the rural health facilities in the survey was linked with the sampled rural PSUs. Primary Health Centres (PHCs) and Sub-Centres in proximity, which catered to the healthcare needs of the sampled rural PSUs, were included in the facility survey. All Community Health Centres and District Hospitals were included in the survey. The reference period for the study was from January to December 2018. The research team visited all the districts and facilities with the detailed questionnaires to collect information from the study area.

Description of the Study Area and Profile

Site Description

The districts located in the northern Bihar are mostly economically backward (Fig. 1.2). Of the surveyed districts, West Champaran is geographically the largest (5228 sq. Km) and has the lowest population density (753 persons/sq. Km), followed by Rohtas (3881 sq. Km in area) with a density of 763 persons/sq. Km. Two of the selected districts—Kishanganj and West Champaran—recorded the highest population growth (30.4 per cent and 30.2 per cent respectively). Rohtas recorded the highest literacy rate (73.4 per cent), while West Champaran (44.6 per cent) and Kishanganj (55.5 per cent) recorded the lowest, the state average being 63.8 per cent. Institutional delivery was the highest in Jehanabad and Rohtas and the lowest in Madhubani and Kishanganj (83.0, 80.7, 50.3, and 41.8 per cent respectively) and deliveries assisted by health personnel were common in high prevalence districts.

The allocation of the health infrastructure was found skewed in the surveyed districts. Evidence of the higher shortage of PHCs about 60 per cent in West Champaran and Rohtas, and more than 70 per cent shortfall of doctors in Kishanganj and Madhubani abundantly available from government sources themselves, that is, from the State Health Society of Bihar.

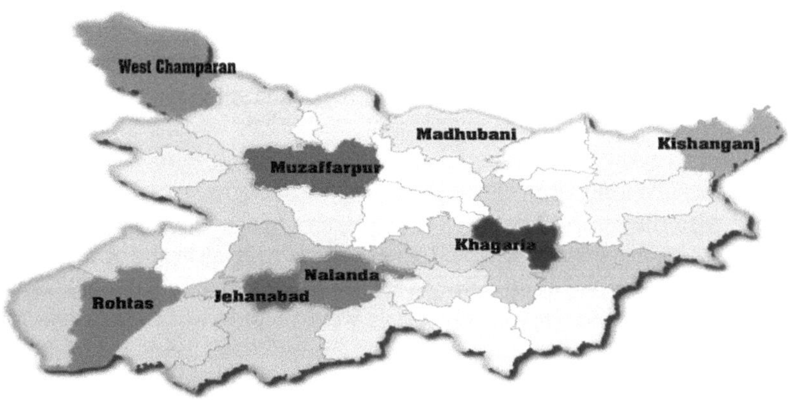

Fig. 1.2 Map of study area

Profile of the Households and Eligible Women Surveyed

The study sample is largely rural-based (90 per cent) and over half of them were from the Other Backward Caste (55 per cent), followed by Scheduled Caste/Tribe (32.4 per cent). The average number of members in a family was five, and most of the families were nuclear in composition. The key earning source of most households was casual labour (52 per cent) in non-agriculture and consists around three-quarters of households in Madhubani, Khagaria, and West Champaran each. The poor economic status of households reflected in their monthly expenditure which is limited only to Rs. 2000/- for more than 85 per cent family. Migration is a common survival strategy for poor households and around in 33 per cent of households, at least one member had migrated for employment with highest proportion in Madhubani. Three in five households relied on and utilised healthcare from private health facilities, despite their poor economic condition. With a low coverage of health insurance (only 11 per cent), households were forced to take loans from either banks or money lenders to meet the treatment cost. Almost one in four respondents lived in kutcha houses, and 33 per cent had a separate cooking space. Almost all households had access to electricity and water within their own premises. However, only a half had a toilet facility and more than 40 per cent used wood/dung as the cooking fuel.

As maternal factors are associated with health of newborn, detailed information on women's biological and social status was collected. In the survey age group 20–29 years comprised 76 per cent of the sample. Most of the sampled population married by age 18 and had limited access to higher education (one in five had attained higher secondary and above levels of education). Female education was relatively better in Rohtas, with approximately 40 per cent having attained higher secondary level of education. Only 6 per cent women were currently engaged as agricultural labourers. The work participation of women was the highest in Nalanda (17 per cent), and it was the lowest in West Champaran (1 per cent).

On an average, women had given birth to less than three children at the time of survey. Around 20 per cent of respondents had more than four children, and 30 per cent had at least one child at the time of the survey. The Parity Progression Ratio (PPR) of women age 30 and above shows that unless PPR at parity 2 or 3 declines significantly, fertility reduction in the state is difficult. This emphasises the significance of family planning measures as it was also observed that unmet need for family planning among the study respondents was almost 12 per cent during the year prior to the survey. The food security and nutritional status of the respondents showed around 23 per cent women were underweight, and a similar per cent faced food insufficiency during pregnancy. More than four-fifths of women surveyed had utilised health services from private facilities. The intra-household decision-making, measured through the women empowerment index, showed a relatively low position (13 per cent) of women in the household, reflecting their lower involvement in healthcare utilisation.

Description of the Surveyed Community (Villages/Wards)

Geographical location of the health centre is determinant to access healthcare, as is evident in the studies. The average distance to the nearest health centre from a village ranges from around 4.5 km in Nalanda and Jehanabad to 10.2 km in Khagaria. Almost all villages had a pucca road, but most of them were inaccessible at the time of floods. Poor drainage facility was most common in the villages of Muzaffarpur and Madhubani. It has been documented that a poor sanitary environment promotes infection and induces stress, especially during the time of pregnancy and delivery (Padhi et al. 2015). Compared to villages, wards had an improved infrastructure in terms of drainage, pucca roads, drinking water, and toilets.

The mid-day meal programme was running in most of the villages. Only around 36 per cent villages were covered by the Integrated Child Development Service (ICDS), with the lowest coverage being in Kishanganj (28.6 per cent). ASHA workers were universally present, but the villages fell short of Auxiliary Nursing Midwifery (ANMs) and doctors. Only 15 per cent villages had a government doctor, and 12 per cent had private qualified practitioners. That made the village people to depend on informal providers. Primary health facilities were found to exist in 40 per cent wards; 30 per cent wards had a government hospital, and half of the wards also had a private hospital/clinic. Functional infrastructure at the facilities was found in Jehanabad and Khagaria. The facilities covered by the study at Kishanganj mostly lacked functional labour rooms, operation theatres, and maternity wards. Waste storage space was mostly missing at the PHC level. The wards surveyed in Madhubani, West Champaran, and Kishanganj did not have any such facilities. One-third of the total wards had an ambulance service. Most of the wards did not have the facility of a 24-hour medical shop.

Diseases like diarrhoea, pneumonia, and jaundice were reported as common ailments among newborns in the community. Lack of proper care was reported as the major reason for death among the newborn in Nalanda and West Champaran. On the contrary, Kishanganj reported absence of any health facility as the primary reason. Socioeconomic differences, low empowerment, poor living conditions, and preference for more children, together with a poor healthcare system, posed major challenges to efforts aimed at improving maternal and child health outcomes in the state.

Overview of the Book

The material presented in the book engages in the exploration of the underlying societal and health system barriers and their interface that jeopardise newborn health. For a comprehensive understanding of the barriers that trigger the risk of death, each chapter deals with specific aspects of maternal and newborn healthcare. The book highlights the status of neonatal mortality across India, the intra-regional inequalities, the facilitators of and barriers to newborn health, and the impact of the interventions and their implications for the health policy.

The first three chapters of the book provide the context to the health of the newborn in Bihar. The first chapter is an introduction to the study, whereby we discuss the rationale behind exploring newborn health, the objectives, in addition to describing the sample design, the study area, and the sample itself. Chapters 2 and 3 analyse the social determinants of neonatal health and provide a direction for understanding newborn health in the regional context of Bihar. The second chapter reviews the literature related to neonatal mortality and unfolds the risk factors in India and the EAG states and the emerging concerns. The chapter is based on the literature review and secondary data analysis. Data drawn from the NFHS, the HMIS, and the SRS was used for the analysis. In Chap. 3, the situation of neonatal health in the specific socio-cultural setting of Bihar is detailed. While doing so, the chapter provides a brief overview of the status of the socioeconomic and health infrastructure to provide the context for why the state was selected. Given the complexity of the environment women live in, this chapter provides insights into newborn health and its differentials across individual, household, and institutional attributes. The chapter draws upon the data collected from the primary investigation and uses the existing secondary information.

The subsequent chapters explore the barriers creating the low care-seeking behaviour vis-à-vis newborn health in Bihar. These chapters examine the process indicators related to mothers and neonates, such as barriers to ANC, facility delivery, quality of facility care, postnatal care, and community-level interventions in bringing about behavioural change. In doing so, the expectations and experiences with regard to the service delivery in the public health system have also been examined. Chapter 4 describes the antenatal care-seeking behaviour and the access to safe delivery services in the study area. Access to antenatal care (ANC) and facility delivery are safe motherhood interventions that reduce maternal and neonatal mortality significantly. Given the low attainment of full ANC and the substantial number of home deliveries in specific pockets of the state, this chapter identifies the socio-structural barriers that emerge from the users' perspective, including norms and cultural beliefs, along with the system-level barriers that shape the access to newborn health services.

Increasing facility delivery without improving quality of services may not translate into reduction in neonatal mortality. Chapter 5 provides an assessment of quality of services received at institutions in terms of both users' satisfaction from the services and the provision of care during the childbirth and hospital stay. While presenting an analysis of quality-of-service delivery, this chapter identifies the gaps in service provision at the facility that will provide directions for further interventions and improve quality of services at facility.

Promoting antenatal care (ANC) and skilled attendance at birth alone may not suffice as the first few hours and days after birth are the riskiest for the newborn and most newborn deaths can be averted through proper care. The knowledge of care and the care practices, however, are influenced by the socio-cultural beliefs, knowledge, and supervision of health workers. Taking these factors into account, Chap. 6 examines the essential practices for newborn care and explores the barriers to them. The purpose of this chapter is to examine the influence of medical, socio-cultural, and economic variables on newborn health through care practices. Community-level interventions are implemented to overcome the demand-side barriers influencing newborn survival. The effectiveness of the home-based newborn care (HBNC) programmes and the role of the community workers in promoting care-seeking practices are hence discussed.

Chapter 7 assesses the results of the above findings in the light of the health infrastructure. Public health infrastructure for newborns, the Sick Newborn Care Units (SNCUs), is critical to shaping healthcare delivery and preventing neonatal death. The enablers of and the barriers to admission in SNCU and the efficiency of SNCU in preventing neonatal mortality are also examined.

A critical assessment of the status and challenges of the existing demand-side financial interventions has been made in Chap. 8. Such interventions are introduced to increase the access to maternal and newborn care services and improve health outcomes. An assessment is made of Direct Benefit Transfer (DBT) schemes, such as Janani Bal Suraksha Yojana (JBSY) and Pradhan Mantri Matru Vandana Yojana (PMMVY), aimed at promoting institutional delivery, influencing neonatal health, and providing financial protection. The implementation challenges are discussed as well.

Chapter 9 discusses the key findings of the study and spells out the policy recommendations for preventing the barriers that trigger neonatal death in the state. Considering the key findings, a note on the way forward is presented, highlighting the critical areas for further investigation, the good practices that need to be followed, and the strategic solutions for accomplishing the targets of Sustainable Development Goals. While providing a way forward for future research and policy action, the need for innovative strategies to be developed for scaling up Maternal Newborn Child Health (MNCH) services and improving neonatal outcomes is discussed.

It is hoped that the key information as well as the recommendations, provided in the book, will broaden the understanding of the pathways of newborn survival in resource-poor settings. It is also believed that the findings of the book will stimulate more discussion and provide guidance for implementing programmes and policies for improving the newborn health situation in resource-poor regions.

References

Arokiasamy, P., & Gautam, A. (2008). Neonatal mortality in the empowered action group states of India: trends and determinants. *Journal of Biosocial Science*, *40*(2), 183–201.

Bora, J. K., & Saikia, N. (2018). Neonatal and under-five mortality rate in Indian districts with reference to Sustainable Development Goal 3: An analysis of the National Family Health Survey of India (NFHS), 2015–2016. *PLoS One*, 13(7): e0201125.

Cleland, J. (2001). The effects of improved survival on fertility: A reassessment. *Population and Development Review*, *27*, 60–92.

Fadel, S. A., Ram, U., Morris, S. K., Begum, R., Shet, A., Jotkar, R., & Jha, P. (2015). Facility delivery, postnatal care and neonatal deaths in India: nationally-representative case-control studies. *PLoS One*, *10*(10), e0140448.

Hochbaum, G., Rosenstock, I., & Kegels, S. (1952). *Health belief model*. United States Public Health Service, 1.

Hug, L., Alexander, M., You, D., Alkema, L., & for Child, U. I. A. G. (2019). National, regional, and global levels and trends in neonatal mortality between 1990 and 2017, with scenario-based projections to 2030: a systematic analysis. *The Lancet Global Health*, *7*(6), e710–e720.

Kapoor, M., Kim, R., Sahoo, T., Roy, A., Ravi, S., Kumar, A. S., ... & Subramanian, S. V. (2020). Association of maternal history of neonatal death with subsequent neonatal death in India. *JAMA Network Open*, *3*(4), e202887–e202887.

Lawn, J., Shibuya, K., & Stein, C. (2005). No cry at birth: global estimates of intrapartum stillbirths and intrapartum-related neonatal deaths. *Bulletin of the World Health Organization*, *83*, 409–417.

Loke, A. Y., Davies, L., & Li, S. F. (2015). Factors influencing the decision that women make on their mode of delivery: the Health Belief Model. *BMC Health Services Research*, *15*(1), 1–12.

Mosley, W. H., & Chen, L. C. (1984). An analytical framework for the study of child survival in developing countries. *Population and Development Review*, *10*, 25–45.

National Health Policy (2002). https://www.india.gov.in/national-health-policy-2002-0

National Population Policy (2000). Dept. of Family Welfare, Ministry of Health and Family Welfare, Government of India.

Neogi, S. B., Pandey, S., Sharma, J., Chokshi, M., Chauhan, M., Zodpey, S., & Paul, V. K. (2015). Association between household air pollution and neonatal mortality: an analysis of Annual Health Survey results, India. *WHO South-East Asia Journal of Public Health*, *4*(1), 30-37.

National Family Health Survey (2015–2016). http://rchiips.org/nfhs/Report_NFHS-4.shtml.

Padhi, B. K., Baker, K. K., Dutta, A., Cumming, O., Freeman, M. C., Satpathy, R., ... &Panigrahi, P. (2015). Risk of adverse pregnancy outcomes among women practicing poor sanitation in rural India: a population-based prospective cohort study. *PLoS Medicine*, *12*(7), e1001851.

Ranganathan, S., Bali Swain, R., & Sumpter, D. J. (2015). *The demographic transition and economic growth: a dynamical systems model*. Palgrave Communications, 1.

Sankar, M. J., Neogi, S. B., Sharma, J., Chauhan, M., Srivastava, R., Prabhakar, P. K., ..., Paul, V. K. (2016). State of newborn health in India. *Journal of Perinatology*, *36*(3), S3–S8.

Srinivasan, K. (2017). *Population concerns in India: shifting trends, policies, and programs*. SAGE Publishing India.
Sample Registration System (2018). https://censusindia.gov.in/vital_statistics/SRS_Reports_2018.html
Suzuki, E., & Kashiwase, H. (2020). https://blogs.worldbank.org/opendata/new-child-and-youth-mortality-estimates-show-dramatic-reductions-progress-threatened
Tinker, A., ten Hoope-Bender, P., Azfar, S., Bustreo, F., & Bell, R. (2005). A continuum of care to save newborn lives. *The Lancet*, *365*(9462), 822–825.
Tymicki, K. (2009). Correlates of infant and childhood mortality: A theoretical overview and new evidence from the analysis of longitudinal data of the Bejsce (Poland) parish register reconstitution study of the 18th–20th centuries. *Demographic Research*, *20*, 559–594.
UNICEF (2014). *Committing to Child Survival: A Promise Renewed.*
UNICEF (2018). The neonatal period is the most vulnerable time for a child. https://data.unicef.org/topic/child-survival/neonatal-mortality
UN IGME (2017). "Levels and Trends in Child Mortality" estimates by UN Inter-agency Group for Child Mortality Estimation.
UN IGME (2019). "Levels and Trends in Child Mortality" estimates by UN Inter-agency Group for Child Mortality Estimation.
World Health Organisation (2020). https://www.who.int/news-room/fact-sheets/detail/newborns-reducing-mortality. https://childmortality.org/files_v21/download/IGME%20report%202017%20child%20mortality%20final.pdf

CHAPTER 2

Determinants of Newborn Survival in India

Introduction

The Convention on Rights of Child ratified in 1989 recognises 'The right of the child[1] *to the enjoyment of the highest attainable standard of health and to facilities for the treatment of illness and rehabilitation of health. State should strive to ensure that no child is deprived of his or her right of access to such healthcare services'.* (UN General Assembly 1989)

Ensuring children's survival and well-being is a national priority as improved health outcomes of children have great familial and societal benefits. Reduction of infant and child mortality also plays a fundamental role in triggering the demographic transition (Pozzi and Fariñas 2015), although historical shreds of evidence do not support the idea that mortality decline accounts for population decline. With the industrial revolution and technological progress, developed countries experienced a fast reduction in mortality (Galor and Weil 2000). Changes in the economic structure, social development, and the process of modernisation have influenced parents to shift from quantity to quality children, which has lowered infant and neonatal mortality in such countries. The less developed countries, on the contrary, have been experiencing a slower decline in the pace of mortality among infants. Although neonatal mortality has been declining in the recent decades, the rate of decrease has been much slower in these

[1] Child means every human being below the age of 18 years.

S. R. Mahapatro, *Towards Newborn Survival*,
https://doi.org/10.1007/978-981-19-3417-9_2

countries. The largest number of neonatal deaths in absolute numbers occurs in the South Asian countries, but the death rate is higher in sub-Saharan Africa. According to the UNICEF (2018), West and Central African countries represented the world's highest neonatal mortality rate in 2015, with an estimate of 31.4 deaths per 1000 live births, followed by the South Asian countries, with 28.9 deaths per 1000 live births. India is the epicentre of neonatal mortality, with every fourth neonate in the world who dies being from India (Lawn et al. 2014). Neonatal Mortality Rate is a key outcome indicator that directly reflects prenatal, intrapartum, and neonatal care and is also a measure of socioeconomic development. The mortality rate of infants and under-five age children decreases with an improvement in newborn survival. Using the data from the Sample Registration System (SRS) and the National Family Health Survey (NFHS), this chapter presents the status and determinants of neonatal mortality in India and its regions. The first section focuses on the trends in neonatal mortality in India, while the second one deals with the risk factors of neonatal death. The observations drawn from this chapter will set the context for the rest of the chapters of the book.

Trends in Neonatal Mortality

India has historically experienced high infant and child mortality. The infant mortality rate (IMR) was unacceptably high till the 1970s and varied between 130 and 140 per 1000 live births. With the turn of the twentieth century, the IMR began to decline at a faster rate, several decades after the mortality transition had begun. Currently, infant mortality is at 32 per 1000 live births (SRS 2018). Figure 2.1 shows the trends in infant, newborn, and post-neonatal mortality rates in India. The two stages of the infant period, that is, neonatal and postnatal, combinedly contribute to infant deaths. The NMR was 75 in 1971 and declined to 23 per 1000 live births in 2018. The post-neonatal mortality rate, which stood at 54 per 1000 live births, dropped to 9 per 1000 live births during this period. According to the SRS, neonatal deaths accounted for 58 per cent of infant deaths in 1971, but increased to 72 per cent in 2018. Conversely, post-neonatal mortality declined from 42 per cent in 1971 to 28 per cent in 2018. The mortality estimates from the different rounds of the NFHS corroborate this finding. The NMR was 49, 43, 39, and 30 per 1000 live births in 1992, 1998, 2005, and 2015 over the five years preceding the respective survey dates. Neonatal deaths as a proportion of infant deaths

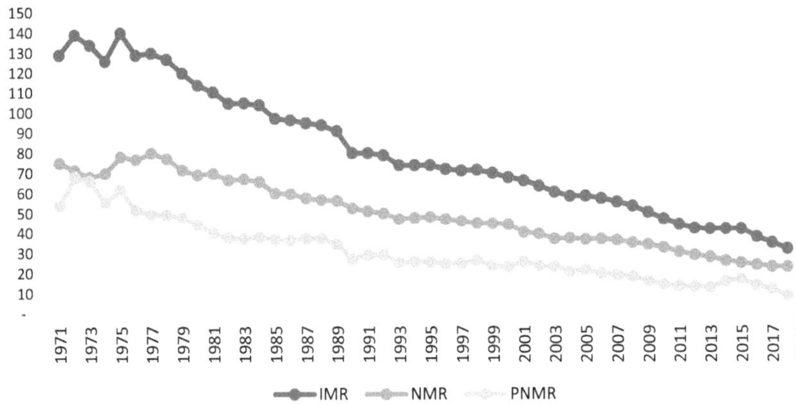

Fig. 2.1 Trends in infant, neonatal, and post-neonatal mortality rates. (Source: SRS 1971–2018)

were 62 per cent during NFHS-1. The share increased continuously to 63 per cent, 68 per cent, and 73 per cent in NFHS-2, NFHS-3, and NFHS-4, respectively. Such results demonstrate that the decline observed in infant mortality is mainly due to a reduction in post-neonatal mortality. In recent years, the decline in NMR has thus been of particular concern.

India has witnessed a significant improvement in neonatal health in recent years with serious efforts by central and state governments. Notwithstanding the focus on neonatal health, the annual rate of reduction in neonatal mortality still lags the IMR and the U5MR. With current trends, India is unlikely to achieve the Sustainable Development Goal target of 12 per 1000 live births by 2030 or the National Health Policy-2025 target of 16 per 1000 live births by 2025 (Dandona et al. 2020). An investigation into the risk factors impacting neonatal mortality is, hence, crucial to formulate an appropriate policy intervention.

Determinants of Neonatal Mortality

Mosley and Chen's (1984) framework has been widely applied in studies aimed at understanding child survival, highlighting the role of socioeconomic, environmental, and biological factors. Globally, studies based on the framework have subsumed the contextual aspects of newborn survival. Neonatal deaths are often incorporated into the more widely used indicators of infant and child mortality, although the factors determining decomposed mortality indicators, such as neonatal, post-neonatal, and child mortality, vary substantially (Arokiasamy and Gautam 2008). Neonatal mortality has been understudied because of three leading reasons: Lack of historical data, underestimation of neonatal deaths that occur during home deliveries, and misreporting of neonatal deaths as stillbirth (Aleshina and Redmond 2005; Målqvist 2011). While realising the role of newborn survival in reducing child mortality, research studies carried out in recent years have found that biomedical, maternal, and socioeconomic conditions are significant risk factors of mortality among the newborns (WHO 2016; Sankar et al. 2016). In poor socio-cultural settings, alongside the challenges of service delivery, cultural and social characteristics, norms, and practices also influence the maternal and newborn health (MNH) and health-seeking behaviour (Caldwell 1990; Bandyopadhyay and MacPherson 1998), which have not been studied well enough. Therefore, exploring the complex interplay of the socio-structural barriers impacting newborn health is key to improve newborn survival.

Demand-Side Factors Associated with Neonatal Mortality

The demand-side adversities that influence health of neonates include variables related to socioeconomic conditions such as caste of household, parental education, household income, and environment and demographic characteristics of mother and family of newborn.

Social Class

The influence of social inequalities on poor health outcomes is evident from numerous studies. Caste, class, race, ethnicity, and gender are the various categories of social hierarchy and differentiation in many societies. The caste system in India is a paradigmatic example of a social hierarchy where an individual is identified based on their caste. Berreman (1967, p. 70) defined the caste system as a 'system of birth-ascribed stratification, of socio cultural pluralism, and hierarchical interaction'. According to the social hierarchy of India, there are four caste groups, namely Scheduled Castes, Scheduled Tribes, Other Backward Classes, and General. Scheduled

Castes/Scheduled Tribes are at the bottom of the social hierarchy. Deprived of developmental opportunities, they take the burden of mortality more than those in the upper social class. While a decline in neonatal mortality is noticed in recent years, there is a heterogeneity in the pattern of decrease, with a higher concentration of deaths among low castes and tribes (Subramanian et al. 2006; Das et al. 2000), mainly due to a lower utilisation of services (Hazarika 2011). The interaction of low social status with multiple vulnerabilities that operate at the household and community levels exacerbates the likelihood of infant and neonatal mortality (Ram et al. 2016). Even though several initiatives have been taken to reduce caste inequalities, there is still a high variability in neonatal health outcomes. Low affordability, accompanied by the remoteness of health centres, lack of health knowledge, cultural practices, and discrimination poses challenges for the more inferior caste women in utilising healthcare in the continuum from pregnancy to the postnatal period.

Parental Education

Extant literature shows a direct association of maternal education with the survival of neonates with high maternal education being associated with an improved status and better access to health information. Since there is a great deal of maternal involvement in child care practices, maternal education greatly influences the choice and skill of care practices. Despite non-accessibility to modern healthcare services, child survival is more remarkable in areas where mothers' level of education is higher (Orubuloye and Caldwell 1975; Yunis et al. 2003). An educated mother makes a swift decision and visits a healthcare facility immediately in the event of ill health, whereas an illiterate mother lacks the capability to do so (Caldwell 1990). Such mothers tend to rely on traditional practices for childbirth and care. Education as a behavioural change intervention improves healthcare utilisation and, thus, the survival of newborns. Cleland (1990) states:

> [E]ducation may have a modest effect on health knowledge and beliefs, but a pronounced effect on the propensity to use modern medical facilities, and adopt modern health practices, because of a closer social identification with the modern world, greater confidence at handling bureaucracies or a more innovative attitude to life among women who have some experience of school.

Household Deprivations

There is convincing evidence that a household's monetary and non-monetary resources are associated with the survival status of the children. Low capacity to pay, intertwined with high cost of services and other vulnerabilities, affects newborn health. A study on neonatal health in the states of Rajasthan, Bihar, and Odisha found that neonatal mortality was higher among the economically poor households as financial and geographical barriers affected their healthcare utilisation (Dogra et al. 2015). Linking poverty and mortality, studies show that several risk factors during the antenatal and neonatal periods—acting through the economic condition, household environment, and nutritional deprivation—affect neonatal health (Wagstaff 2002). Housing characteristics such as access to safe drinking water, hygiene practices, and clean cooking fuel have a positive influence on newborn survival, with a reduction in the risk of infection and diarrhoeal diseases (Neogi et al. 2015; Lakshmi et al. 2013). Though childbirth is a joyous occasion, mother and newborn are considered impure for some period in many parts of the country. Therefore, they are kept in an isolated place, with the period of seclusion varying according to caste, class, and religion. Such practices, based on the belief of the theory of purity and pollution, affect the postnatal care of newborn and mother (Bandyopadhyay and MacPherson 1998).

Demographic Factors

The demographic characteristics of mother and child, such as lower birth interval, birth order, birth size, or maternal age, have been acknowledged as the proximate determinants of child survival (Titaley et al. 2008; Saugstad 2011). These are mainly the endogenous factors, biological in nature, related to some impairment during the formation of the foetus in the womb and other cognitive or neurological deformities inside the womb. For instance, low birth weight babies may result from premature births, which could predispose them to infections and other abnormalities (Lawn and Kerber 2006). On the other hand, larger babies have a higher risk of birth injury, respiratory distress due to birth asphyxia, and congenital anomalies, exposing them to a higher likelihood of neonatal death (Ng et al. 2010). Gender of the child is also an important predictor, with a higher mortality among boys than girls, mainly due to immunodeficiency leaving baby boys more vulnerable to infectious diseases (Arokiasamy and Gautam 2008), resulting, therefore, in a higher prevalence of respiratory diseases in males and congenital malformations of the urogenital system.

Supply of Health Services and Neonatal Mortality

Access to and utilisation of neonatal healthcare services influence newborn survival considerably (Frankenberg 1995). Regular antenatal care visits provide an opportunity to educate women about preventive care—such as by providing counselling on breastfeeding, hygiene, nutrition, and early identification of pregnancy complications—that increases the chances of survival and promotes the well-being of neonates (Mahmood 2002). The use of ANC serves as a facilitating platform linking the woman and her family to the healthcare system, which significantly affects newborn and child health (Dixit et al. 2013). ANC's impact on neonatal survival though not observed in some studies (Mbuagbaw et al. 2015), a majority of the studies suggest it is a fundamental preventive strategy to reduce the risk of neonatal mortality (WHO 2016; Singh et al. 2013; Rammohan et al. 2013). In resource-poor places like Nigeria, sub-Saharan Africa, and Ethiopia, being born to women who have not made ANC visits increases the chances of neonatal deaths. These mothers are devoid of information related to newborn care practices and early detection of complications and have lower chances of delivering the baby through skilled birth attendants (SBAs) (Amouzou et al. 2017).

Place of delivery often determines the quality of care—such as sanitary environment and medically correct birth assistance during delivery—and, hence, is likely to reduce newborn deaths (Ajaari et al. 2012). The presence of SBAs, either medical doctors, nurses, or midwives, is essential to ensure appropriate management of the delivery process and prevent fatal events attributed to delivery-related complications (WHO 2005). To add to the benefits, it is seen that the combination of facility delivery and postnatal check-ups during the neonatal period has a protective effect on newborn survival (Lawn and Kerber 2006; Sines et al. 2007) as it allows for supervision by medical personnel in terms of healthy breastfeeding, identification of a critical illness, and growth monitoring of newborns.

Health education is an important indicator of maternal and newborn healthcare utilisation in India. Studies find that lack of awareness and cultural beliefs play a vital role in influencing maternal and child health-seeking behaviour (Kumar et al. 2015; Awasthi 2011). Self-belief, convenience, and family pressure are cited as reasons for cultural practices (Shekar and Babu 2009). To overcome various demand-side challenges, innovative strategies—such as JBSY, PMMVY, JSSK, and HBNC—have been implemented over time in the country. Conditional cash transfers have been implemented to promote institutional delivery and improve health outcomes. Community-based interventions in various parts of India show that home-based essential newborn care and health education are associated with reduced neonatal mortality (Bang et al. 2005). However, the effective implementation of such programmes is constrained by the weak health system and the challenging contextual factors, including socio-cultural and gender-based barriers (Lunze et al. 2015). A study by Awasthi (2011) in Lucknow, Uttar Pradesh, found that modern health practices were less acceptable, quacks were trusted, and harmful cultural practices overrode authentic practices mainly due to the lack of awareness about their potential harm. This raises an important question as to how far the demand-side interventions of the health system address the barriers to service utilisation and contribute to improving newborn health outcomes.

In India, the maternal and newborn health outcomes vary across the states, which are accordingly classified as EAG and Non-EAG states. Availability, acceptability, and affordability are three elements that influence access to MNCH services. There persists a large regional disparity in health infrastructure, with a skewed allocation of physical and human resources, including quality of service. The deficiency of services is particularly pronounced in the EAG states, namely Bihar, Madhya Pradesh, Uttar Pradesh, Chhattisgarh, Jharkhand, Odisha, and Rajasthan. Access to affordable and quality health infrastructure positively influences people's health status (Baru et al. 2010; Saikia and Das 2016). The impact of socio-economic development on health infrastructure has been evident from studies (Mahapatro and Singh 2016). Most studies have, so far, focused on infant and child mortality, paying limited attention to neonatal health. It is important to identify the underlying risk factors of newborn survival in India, especially so, in the EAG states.

Identification of Risk Factors of Newborn Survival: Results from Probit Analysis

I used the multivariate probit regression model separately for India and the EAG states to analyse the effect of social determinants on neonatal mortality. The birth history of a surviving mother during five years prior to the date of the NFHS-4 survey was used. A separate analysis for the EAG states was done as these states account for nearly half of the population and perform poorly on maternal and newborn health indicators.

The statistical analysis confirmed the earlier literature discussed on the risk factors of newborn survival. Birth size, lower birth interval, higher birth order, and younger or older maternal age were associated with a higher likelihood of neonatal mortality. On the other hand, antenatal care, facility delivery by health professionals, and maternal education had a protective effect against neonatal mortality. Infants born in less affluent and marginalised communities in resource-poor states experience a high NMR. Limited capacity to spend on healthcare, followed by unhygienic living conditions, poor sanitation, and discriminatory practices by providers expose the newborns to infectious diseases and lower their chances of survival. Infants delivered by mothers in the EAG states had a higher likelihood of death. These resource-poor states face the challenge of poor health infrastructure. Cultural attitudes, socioeconomic backwardness, and low status of women in these states affect the use of healthcare.

Unlike the all-India analysis, the analysis for the EAG states did not show much impact of mother's education on neonatal health as only the primary level of education was associated with it. Perhaps this is because the patriarchal family relationship and the lower status of women in these states do not allow women to seek healthcare of their choice. Most of the EAG states are out-migrating states from where males migrate to other states for employment. In many instances, the absence of the husband likely creates obstacles to accessing healthcare for mother and newborn despite the mother having an education. Another variation between India as a whole and the EAG states was found in C-section deaths, with neonatal deaths being higher in the EAG states. This indicates that delay in access to healthcare or negligence on the part of the providers at a facility can cause higher deaths among newborns. Within the EAG states, Uttar Pradesh and Chhattisgarh had a higher likelihood of neonatal deaths.

Discussion

The results drawn from this chapter provide a set of socio-demographic risk factors of newborn survival. The demographic transition, that is underway across the globe, shows that the decline in mortality became faster in the early 1930s with the control of famines and epidemics, much before the medical interventions became available. This underlies the significance of socio-demographic and cultural factors in determining the health of infants and children.

The analysis, however, has certain limitations that need to be considered for a deeper understanding of newborn health. First, most of the literature analyses trends and determinants relating mainly to infant and under-five mortality and extends them to neonatal health. Furthermore, the available literature on NMR focuses only on the determinants of neonatal mortality. A comprehensive assessment of newborn health from continuum of care perspective has not been made in any Indian study. Secondly, the analysis based on the existing data sources emphasises on the characteristics of the users and the associated risk factors of newborn health. Apart from socioeconomic and biological conditions, supply-side challenges also pose as barriers to newborn health. The existing data sets have limitations in how much and how well they can address the supply-side challenges and community-led interventions to bring about behavioural change and, in turn, increase service utilisation. The analysis does not emphasise the role of postnatal care practices that a newborn receives both in the hospital and at home during 28 days. Thirdly, no detailed, systematic investigation has been done into the factors contributing to regional variability in neonatal mortality. The present analysis and the previous studies done in India have found a noticeable regional disparity in neonatal mortality. The localised diversities that vary across the states act as obstacles to the use of services and, hence, to newborn survival.

While few states of India are comparable to the best-performing nations of the Asian region, we have many states whose performance is lower than that of many less developed countries, and Bihar is one among them. A blanket approach to reducing neonatal mortality within the EAG states may not be the best option in this context. The structural conditions, the political ideologies, and the developmental approaches of a particular state government, interacting with the personal variables, culture, norms, and so on, influence health outcomes. Indeed, a micro-level inquiry into the underlying mechanisms influencing newborn survival will provide a better understanding of the contextual barriers to newborn health. This will allow policymakers to design potential interventions to address neonatal death accordingly. The next chapter will address the newborn health with a regional perspective.

References

Ajaari, J., Masanja, H., Weiner, R., Abokyi, S. A., & Owusu-Agyei, S. (2012). Impact of place of delivery on neonatal mortality in rural Tanzania. *International Journal of MCH and AIDS*, *1*(1), 49.

Aleshina, N., & Redmond, G. (2005). How high is infant mortality in Central and Eastern Europe and the Commonwealth of Independent States?. *Population Studies*, *59*(1), 39–54.

Amouzou, A., Ziqi, M., Carvajal-Aguirre, L., &Quinley, J. (2017). Skilled attendant at birth and newborn survival in Sub–Saharan Africa. *Journal of Global Health*, *7*(2).

Arokiasamy, P., & Gautam, A. (2008). Neonatal mortality in the empowered action group states of India: trends and determinants. *Journal of Biosocial Science*, *40*(2), 183–201.

Awasthi, A. (2011). Role of awareness and education to reduce child mortality. *Voice of Intellectual Man-An International Journal*, *1*(1), 129–134.

Bandyopadhyay, M., & MacPherson, S. (1998). *Women and Health: Tradition and Culture in Rural India: Tradition and Culture in Rural India*. Routledge.

Bang, A. T., Bang, R. A., Reddy, H. M., Deshmukh, M. D., & Baitule, S. B. (2005). Reduced incidence of neonatal morbidities: effect of home-based neonatal care in rural Gadchiroli, India. *Journal of Perinatology*, *25*(1), S51–S61.

Baru, R., Acharya, A., Acharya, S., Kumar, A. S., & Nagaraj, K. (2010). Inequities in access to health services in India: caste, class and region. *Economic and Political Weekly*, 49–58.

Berreman, G. D. (1967). Caste as social process. *Southwestern Journal of Anthropology*, *23*(4), 351–370.

Caldwell, J. C. (1990). *Mass education as a determinant of mortality decline*. Center for Advanced Study of International Development, Michigan State University.

Cleland, J.G. (1990). Maternal education and child survival: Further evidence and explanations. In *What we know about the health transition: The cultural, social and behavioural determinants of health, Vol. I*, eds. J. Caldwell, S. Findley, P. Caldwell, G. Santow, J. Braid and D. Broers-Freeman (pp. 400–19) Canberra: Health Transition Centre, The Australian National University

Dandona, R., Kumar, G. A., Henry, N. J., Joshua, V., Ramji, S., Gupta, S. S., … Dandona, L. (2020). Subnational mapping of under-5 and neonatal mortality trends in India: The Global Burden of Disease Study 2000–17. *The Lancet*, *395*(10237), 1640–1658.

Das, N. P., Bhavsar, S., & Patel, R. (2000). *The growth and development of scheduled caste and scheduled tribe population in Gujarat and future prospects.* Population Research Centre, Department of Statistics, Faculty of Science [MS University of Baroda].

Dixit, P., Dwivedi, L. K., & Ram, F. (2013). Strategies to improve child immunization via antenatal care visits in India: a propensity score matching analysis. *PloS One*, *8*(6), e66175

Dogra, V., Khanna, R., Jain, A., Kumar, A. M., Shewade, H. D., & Majumdar, S. S. (2015). Neonatal mortality in India's rural poor: Findings of a household survey and verbal autopsy study in Rajasthan, Bihar and Odisha. *Journal of Tropical Pediatrics*, *61*(3), 210–214.

Frankenberg, E. (1995). The effects of access to health care on infant mortality in Indonesia. *Health Transition Review*, 143–163.

Galor, O., & Weil, D. N. (2000). Population, technology, and growth: From Malthusian stagnation to the demographic transition and beyond. *American Economic Review*, *90*(4), 806–828.

Hazarika, I. (2011). Factors that determine the use of skilled care during delivery in India: implications for achievement of MDG-5 targets. *Maternal and Child Health Journal*, *15*(8), 1381–1388.

Kumar, A., Unnikrishnan, B., Rekha, T., Mithra, P., Kumar, N., Kulkarni, V., & Ramesh Holla, D. B. (2015). Awareness and attitude regarding breastfeeding and immunization practices among primigravida attending a tertiary care hospital in Southern India. *Journal of Clinical and Diagnostic Research: JCDR*, *9*(3), LC01.

Lakshmi, P. V. M., Virdi, N. K., Sharma, A., Tripathy, J. P., Smith, K. R., Bates, M. N., & Kumar, R. (2013). Household air pollution and stillbirths in India: analysis of the DLHS-II National Survey. *Environmental Research*, *121*, 17–22.

Lawn, J., & Kerber, K. (2006). *Opportunities for Africa's Newborns: Practical data, policy and programmatic support for newborn care in Africa*. Partnership for Maternal, Newborn and Child Health, Cape Town, 32.

Lawn, J. E., Blencowe, H., Oza, S., You, D., Lee, A. C., Waiswa, P., ... Lancet Every Newborn Study Group. (2014). Every Newborn: progress, priorities, and potential beyond survival. *The Lancet*, *384*(9938), 189–205.

Lunze, K., Higgins-Steele, A., Simen-Kapeu, A., Vesel, L., Kim, J., & Dickson, K. (2015). Innovative approaches for improving maternal and newborn health-a landscape analysis. *BMC Pregnancy and Childbirth*, *15*(1), 1–19.

Mahapatro, S. R., & Singh, Y. (2016). Response of Health Outcomes to Health Infrastructure: Evidence from Bihar and Tamil Nadu. *ArthaVijnana: Journal of The Gokhale Institute of Politics and Economics*, *58*(4), 349–364.

Mahmood, M. A. (2002). Determinants of neonatal and post-neonatal mortality in Pakistan. *The Pakistan Development Review*, 723–744.

Målqvist, M. (2011). Neonatal mortality: an invisible and marginalised trauma. *Global Health Action*, *4*(1), 5724.

Mbuagbaw, L., Medley, N., Darzi, A. J., Richardson, M., Garga, K. H., &Ongolo-Zogo, P. (2015). Health system and community level interventions for improving antenatal care coverage and health outcomes. *Cochrane Database of Systematic Reviews*, (12).

Mosley, W. H., & Chen, L. C. (1984). An analytical framework for the study of child survival in developing countries. *Population and Development Review, 10*, 25–45.

Neogi, S. B., Pandey, S., Sharma, J., Chokshi, M., Chauhan, M., Zodpey, S., & Paul, V. K. (2015). Association between household air pollution and neonatal mortality: an analysis of Annual Health Survey results, India. *WHO South-East Asia Journal of Public Health, 4*(1), 30–37.

Ng, S. K., Olog, A., Spinks, A. B., Cameron, C. M., Searle, J., & McClure, R. J. (2010). Risk factors and obstetric complications of large for gestational age births with adjustments for community effects: results from a new cohort study. *BMC Public Health, 10*(1), 1–10.

Orubuloye, I. O., & Caldwell, J. C. (1975). The impact of public health services on mortality: a study of mortality differentials in a rural area of Nigeria. *Population Studies, 29*(2), 259–272.

Pozzi, L., &Fariñas, D. R. (2015). Infant and child mortality in the past. In *Annales de démographiehistorique* (No. 1, pp. 55–75). Belin.

Ram, B., Singh, A., & Yadav, A. (2016). The persistent caste divide in India's infant mortality: A study of Dalits (ex-untouchables), Adivasis (indigenous peoples), Other Backward Classes, and forward castes. *Canadian Studies in Population [ARCHIVES], 43*(3–4), 249–63.

Rammohan, A., Iqbal, K., & Awofeso, N. (2013). Reducing neonatal mortality in India: Critical role of access to emergency obstetric care. Baradaran HR, editor. *PLoS One, 8*: e57244.

Saikia, D., & Das, K. K. (2016). Access to public health-care in the rural north-east India.

Sankar, M. J., Neogi, S. B., Sharma, J., Chauhan, M., Srivastava, R., Prabhakar, P. K., … Paul, V. K. (2016). State of newborn health in India. *Journal of Perinatology, 36*(3), S3–S8.

Saugstad, O. D. (2011). Reducing global neonatal mortality is possible. *Neonatology, 99*(4), 250–257.

Shekar, C., & Babu, R. (2009). Cultural factors in health and oral health. *Indian Journal of Dental Advancements, 1*(1), 24–30.

Sines, E., Syed, U., Wall, S., & Worley, H. (2007). Postnatal care: A critical opportunity to save mothers and newborns. *Policy Perspectives on Newborn Health, 1*(7).

Singh, A., Kumar, A., & Kumar, A. (2013). Determinants of neonatal mortality in rural India, 2007–2008. *PeerJ, 1*, e75.

SRS (2018). https://censusindia.gov.in/vital_statistics/SRS_Reports_2018.html

Subramanian, S. V., Nandy, S., Irving, M., Gordon, D., Lambert, H., & Davey Smith, G. (2006). The mortality divide in India: the differential contributions of gender, caste, and standard of living across the life course. *American Journal of Public Health, 96*(5), 818–825.

Titaley, C. R., Dibley, M. J., Agho, K., Roberts, C. L., & Hall, J. (2008). Determinants of neonatal mortality in Indonesia. *BMC Public Health, 8*(1), 1–15.

Assembly, U. G. (1989). Convention on the Rights of the Child. *United Nations, Treaty Series, 1577*(3), 1–23.

UNICEF (2018). https://data.unicef.org/topic/child-survival/neonatal-mortality.

Wagstaff, A. (2002). Inequality aversion, health inequalities and health achievement. *Journal of Health Economics, 21*(4), 627–641.

World Health Organization. (2016). *WHO recommendations on antenatal care for a positive pregnancy experience*. World Health Organization.

World Health Organization. (2005). *The World health report: 2005: make every mother and child count*. World Health Organization.

Yunis, K., Beydoun, H., Khogali, M., Alameh, M., & Tamim, H. (2003). Low socioeconomic status and neonatal outcomes in an urban population in a developing country. *The Journal of Maternal-Fetal & Neonatal Medicine, 14*(5), 338–343.

CHAPTER 3

Neonatal Mortality in Bihar: Critical Reflections

Introduction

We learned in the previous chapter that the NMR in India has been declining but that the progress is uneven across the regions. There is a considerable heterogeneity in neonatal mortality between the demographically progressive states (e.g. Kerala and Tamil Nadu) and those lagging behind (e.g. Bihar and Uttar Pradesh). Southern states—with a well-developed health infrastructure and socioeconomic development, for instance, Kerala and Tamil Nadu—have an NMR of 5 and 10 per 1000 live births respectively. Likewise, Punjab, one of the wealthiest states of the northern region, also has a lower NMR (13 per 1000 live births). Among the major states, Punjab ranks the lowest in terms of percentage share of neonatal death to infant death (61.2 per cent). The highest burden of neonatal mortality is clustered in the central and eastern region, specifically in the EAG states of India. With little more than a modest improvement, the neonatal mortality rates remain unacceptably high in these states. The EAG states of Madhya Pradesh, Uttar Pradesh, Odisha, Rajasthan, Bihar, Jharkhand, and Uttarakhand recorded an NMR of 35, 32, 31, 26, 25, 22, and 21 per 1000 live births respectively in 2018 (SRS 2018).

Many studies on neonatal mortality conducted in India, like in other sub-Saharan Africa and South Asian countries, emphasise on sub-national estimation and focus on the influence of individual-level attributes determining NMR, using secondary data sources. Being based on secondary

S. R. Mahapatro, *Towards Newborn Survival*,
https://doi.org/10.1007/978-981-19-3417-9_3

data sets, uncovering the contextual adversities prevents newborn survival to be limited in those studies. A specific assessment of the state of newborn health with ground-level facts will throw light on the contextual impediments that affect newborn health. The present book makes an attempt to fill this gap by studying Bihar, one of the poorest states of India that consistently records poor health outcomes.

Bihar, the third most populous state of India and characterised as a socioeconomically backward state, has experienced stagnancy in neonatal mortality rates for decades, with a dip only in recent years. We have learned from sociological theories and frameworks that regions with low socioeconomic levels and high-income inequality often have poor health outcomes due to their social, behavioural, and physical environment. In Bihar the intra-regional inequalities in the socioeconomic and healthcare structure possibly influence the neonatal health outcomes. This chapter comes in response to the need to explore in detail the neonatal health situation of Bihar and set the context to analyse the barriers related to newborn care. The first section of the chapter provides an overview of the socioeconomic and health status of the state. This will place Bihar in a larger context to understand its neonatal health situation. The second section of the chapter examines the socioeconomic differentials in NMR as also the use of MNCH services and its association with NMR, using primary data. This section helps understand the local context affecting service utilisation and, hence, neonatal health.

The Economy and the Social System of Bihar

Located in the Eastern Gangetic plains of India, the state of Bihar covers 3 per cent of the geographical spread but 8.6 per cent of the population of the country. It is the third most populous state of India, the population, as of the 2011 census, being 10.4 crore and projected to reach 12.7 crore by 2021. Close to 90 per cent of Bihar's 104.1 million population lives in rural areas. The population density is 1106 persons per sq. km, more than three times higher than the average density of India (382). Administratively, the state is divided into 9 divisions, 38 districts, 101 sub-divisions, and 534 blocks. It is delimited by Nepal in the north, Jharkhand in the south, West Bengal in the east, and Uttar Pradesh in the west.

Bihar has emerged as one of the fastest-growing, low-income Indian states in recent years. Table 3.1 presents the socioeconomic and demographic performance of the state as compared to India. The level of poverty saw a relative downfall from 54.4 per cent in 2004–2005 to 33.7 per cent in 2011–2012. The state is still known to have the largest number

Table 3.1 Socioeconomic conditions, demography, and health outcomes in Bihar and India

Indicators	*Bihar*	*India*	*Source*
Economic			
Per capita (NSDP)	US $640	US $1964	MoSPI, 2020
GSDP growth (at 2011–2012 price)	10.5	6.8	MoSPI, 2018–2019
Percentage below poverty line	33.7	21.9	Planning Commission
Unemployment rate	10	5.8	Periodic Labour Force Survey, NSO, 2018
Social			
Human Development Index	0.576	0.647	India Human Development Report, 2019
Urbanisation	11.3	31.3	Census of India (2011)
Gross enrolment ratio in higher education	14.5	27.0	All India Survey on Higher Education (AISHE) (2019–2020)
Literacy rate	61.8	72.99	Census (2011), Office of Registrar General of India
Women with more than ten years of schooling	22.8	35.7	National Family Health Survey, 2015–2016
Women LFPR (rural)	3.8	23.7	Periodic Labour Force Survey, NSO, 2018
Demography and health			
Decadal population growth	25.4	17.7	Census of India (2011)
Total fertility rate	3.2	2.2	National Family Health Survey, 2015–2016
Maternal mortality ratio	165	122	Sample Registration System, 2015–2017
Life expectancy at birth	69.1	69.4	
Crude birth rate	26.2	20	Sample Registration System (2018)
Crude death rate	6.2	5.8	
Under-five mortality rate	37	36	
Infant mortality rate	32	32	
Neonatal mortality rate	25	23	
Early neonatal mortality rate	20	18	
Population per sub-centre	1067	819	National Health Profile, 2019
Population per PHC	5592	5042	
Population per CHC	70,795	23,080	
Population per public hospital	92,582	50,355	
Population per public hospital bed	9104	1818	
Short fall in sub-centre (%)	58	24	Rural Health Statistics (2019–2020)
Shortfall in PHC (%)	53	29	
Shortfall in CHC (%)	98	38	
PHCS as per IPHS norm (%)	5	13	

living below the poverty line, and the income inequality in the state continues to grow (World Bank 2016). The village economy is mainly agrarian and is based on semi-feudal relations of production that pave the way for class inequalities. The growth trajectories of the state reveal that the average GDP growth rate remained around 5 per cent until 2005. However, the economy has been on the path of continuous growth since, which is perhaps attributable to the shift in the political regime. Recently, the growth rate of Bihar's GSDP was, on average, over 10 per cent higher than the Indian average of 6.8 per cent (Economic Survey 2019–2020). This growth is stimulated by the increase in the public expenditure on infrastructure and social sectors such as health and education. This positive transformation underway in the state is, however, accompanied by a wide intra-regional inequality. As the core develops, drawing resources from the peripheral zones (Bhattacharya 2009), such inequality in the economic growth has led to an increase in inter-state disparities, with districts like Patna, Nalanda, Gaya, Bhagalpur, and Muzaffarpur emerging as centres of growth in the state (Diwakar and Mehendru 2020).

Despite a marked economic growth, more than a third of the state's population lives below the poverty line, and ranked highest in multidimensionally poverty index, recently making the state rank the highest in poverty with a high unemployment rate. According to the 2018–2019 Periodic Labour Force Survey (PLFS), the unemployment rate in Bihar was 10.2 per cent, well above the India average of 5.8 per cent. Agriculture is the mainstay of economy and supports the livelihood of over three-quarters of the population (Bihar Economic Survey 2019–2020). The sector, however, is extremely volatile due to natural disasters—flood in the northern region and drought in the south—that affect the rural household economy. Low levels of industrialisation, absence of sustainable employment opportunities, and an unreliable agriculture, combined with a rising labour demand in the more developed regions, have led to the movement of the young generation, creating a culture of labour migration in the state. The capitalist mode of development increases the demand for casual labour in the more developed states and, hence, a large share of the working-age population of the state has adopted migration as a way of life. Being a labour surplus state, Bihar is a highly out-migrating state after Uttar Pradesh, with migration representing 28 per cent of the total population of the state (Census 2011). The state has the lowest position among all states/UTs in terms of human capital development (0.576), below the national value (0.647). The level of urbanisation is far too low, that is,

11.3 per cent, which is just a little higher than Himachal Pradesh (10 per cent) and has a skewed pattern, varying from 43.1 per cent in the Patna district to 3.5 per cent in the Banka district. Given the environment, it begs the question as to whether the current growth is sustainable and equitable in the state. There is some apprehension when we look at the other social and health indicators of the state.

The social environment of Bihar has been historically marked by caste and class inequalities. The caste system continues to be important for structuring relations of production in agrarian Bihar and makes the state an exception to the changes the Indian society is generally associated with because of the British rule (Chakravarti 2001). The caste composition shows that the scheduled caste population constitutes 15.9 per cent of the total population, which is close to the national average (16.2 per cent), whereas the scheduled tribes constitute a minimal share (1.3 per cent). Within the social system of India, including Bihar, SCs/STs are a socially excluded and marginalised group. The social discrimination, due to their low social status, deprived them of opportunities of development, including healthcare, resulting in a concentration of poor health among them. Alongside a rigid caste system exists a rigid class system based on feudal agrarian class relations. This class-caste continuum is a strong predictor of the ongoing syndrome of poverty and inequality in the state (Prasad and Rodgers 1983; Rodgers 2012). The inhabitants of the state, segregated by religion, show a composition that is more than three-fifth (82.69 per cent) Hindu and 16.87 per cent Muslim.

The low socioeconomic condition of the state is compounded by the low level of literacy. The literacy rate in Bihar has risen steadily over the years and stands at 61.8 per cent, though it is lower than the national average (73 per cent) and the progress has been slower than in many other states. The gross enrolment ratio in higher education is almost half (14.5 per cent) of the Indian average of 27 per cent (All India Survey on Higher Education (AISHE) 2019–2020). The social status of women in the state is relatively low, with early and, even, child marriage being rampant, which strengthens the patriarchal relations in the family. The social status of women, however, is gradually improving with an increasing level of education. The number of women who have ten and more years of schooling has increased (22.8) but remains below the national average (35.7).

Demography and Health Status

Bihar has consistently lagged behind other states of India in respect of the demographic transition, primarily attributed to the sluggish pace of fertility transition that has placed the state right at the top in terms of TFR. Early pregnancy, relatively longer reproductive span, and low birth spacing have resulted in high fertility, which has significant implications for mortality indicators. The annual growth rate of population declined from 2.5 per cent in 1991–2001 to an estimated 1.8 per cent in 2011–2019 (Bihar Economic Survey, 2019–2020) but remains higher than the national average of 1.1 per cent. The reason is that the state has experienced fertility decline with a shift from the pre-transition stage of 5.7 children in the 1980s (SRS) to the mid-transition stage of 3.0 in 2019–2020. Although fertility transition is underway in Bihar, the pace of decline should be hastened as high fertility rate puts a lot of burden on the limited resources.

Poor nutritional status of women has a significant impact on newborn survival as it plays an important role in foetal growth. About one-quarter of women of reproductive age group reported a low BMI and, surprisingly, anaemia during pregnancy increased from 58 per cent to 63 per cent during 2005–2020. More than 40 per cent children of the state were malnourished. The variation in the nutritional status across the districts showed that 26 districts had between 43 and 50 per cent stunted children and nearly 7 districts had the largest number of underweight children. Inter-district data on anaemia among children and adults provided an eye-opening fact on the nutritional deficiency. Although the IMR of Bihar and India are similar, the NMR in the state is above the national average (25 as against 23 per 1000 live births) and contributes to 78 per cent of all infant deaths. While the state of Kerala has already achieved the desired targets of SDGs, the NMR in Bihar is five times that of Kerala. A high NMR forces people to have more children. The state, thus, appears to be in a vicious cycle of high fertility and poor health and nutrition. Table 3.2 presents the glimpses of progress in the MNCH indicators between three rounds of the NFHS.

Access to and utilisation of maternal and child healthcare services have increased significantly over one and half decades. Instances of visiting a healthcare facility within the first trimester of pregnancy increased nearly three-fold, and facility delivery gained importance with an almost four-fold increase between 2005 and 2020. This signifies the programmes implemented for the MNCH services comply with the demand. While infant mortality declined by around 25 per cent, the percentage decline in the NMR was slow during 2005–2020. The district-wise variation in the NMR shows 26 districts have an NMR more than 30 per 1000 live births and, among them, 11 have an NMR more than 40 (Ranjan and Dwivedi 2019). Children who received a health check-up from a doctor/nurse/ ANM, an indicator of early neonatal care, make up only 59.3 per cent. The rate of decline in NMR does not comply with the manifold increase in facility delivery. This implies that facility birth does not confer a survival benefit on neonates in the state. It is needless to mention how formidable a challenge it is posing to the healthcare system. The policy of increasing the coverage of facility birth, without a corresponding improvement in healthcare resources with improved quality, does not appear to succeed in newborn survival. Thus, policies should emphasise on revamping the health system, with a focus on improvement in the quality of care.

Status of Healthcare Resources in the State

Various studies have documented that well-managed public healthcare system plays a critical role in influencing mortality indicators. Unlike the more developed states, the EAG states, specifically UP and Bihar, grapple with an inadequate and inequitable distribution of public health infrastructure. In terms of shortfall of physical infrastructure, Bihar stands next to Uttar Pradesh (Avinash 2020). Currently, rural Bihar has 9112 sub-centres, 1702 PHCs, 57 CHCs, 864 health and wellness centres, 35 sub-divisional hospitals, 36 district hospitals, and 8 medical colleges (Rural Health Statistics 2019–2020). The rural areas of the state are starved of healthcare resources, and the expansion in the size of the health infrastructure has not been satisfactory. For instance, the average population covered per sub-centre, PHC, and CHC was 1067, 5592, and 70,795 respectively, much higher than the aggregate figures of 819, 5042, and 23,080 respectively. Likewise, while 1818 population was served per government hospital bed in India, the figure was almost five times higher in Bihar.

At the aggregate level, the shortfall in SCs, PHCs, and CHCs was 24 per cent, 29 per cent, and 38 per cent in India as a whole, and it stood at 58 per cent, 53 per cent, and 98 per cent respectively in Bihar (Table 3.2). Only 6 per cent PHCs had infrastructure as per Indian Public Health Standard Norms (IPHS) indicating huge shortfall of resources in many dimensions. For instance, less than 30 per cent PHCs functioning 24*7

Table 3.2 Maternal and child health indicators, NFHS-3, NFHS-4, and NFHS-5

Maternal and child health indicators	*NFHS-5 (2019–2020)*	*NFHS-4 (2015–2016)*	*NFHS-3 (2005–2006)*
Percentage of mothers received antenatal care within first trimester	52.9	34.6	18.7
Mothers who had four antenatal visits	25.2	14.4	11.2
Institutional delivery	76.2	63.8	19.9
Home births with SBA	6.1	8.2	9.7
Children received postnatal care within two days after delivery	59.3	–	–
Mothers received postnatal care within two days after delivery	57.3	42.3	13.4
Neonatal mortality	34.5	36.7	39.8
Infant mortality	46.8	48	62
Under-five mortality	56.4	58	85

basis and have at least 4 beds and only one-fifth of PHCs have operation theatre in the state which is much lower than Indian average where more than three-quarter of PHCs performs well in all indicators. While 54,533 population was served per government hospital in Bihar in 2009, the burden had almost doubled to 92,582 in 2018. In 2016, the state had 114 health facilities per 1 million population, which had declined to 99 by 2021 and is projected to decline further to 85 by 2041 given the current pace of improvement (Bihar Economic Survey 2019–2020).

Comparatively, the state has a greater number of PHCs than many EAG states but falls short of ANMs, doctors, beds, and hospitals (National Health Profile 2018). As against the sanctioned posts for 2314 contractual doctors, only 533 posts have been filled up, representing again a high vacancy ratio of 77 per cent (Bihar Economic Survey 2019). As per a WHO recommendation, the doctor-population ratio should be 1:1000. In Bihar, 1 doctor serves 38,000 people, a lot higher than the national average of 11,000. Although the number of required doctors exceeds the requirement per PHC, there is a huge shortfall of specialists in the state. Specialists for the CHCs, pharmacists, and lab technicians are just 14 per cent, 14 per cent, and 30 per cent of the requirement respectively. ASHAs, the backbone of the health system, are overburdened as there is a shortfall of 14 per cent. Furthermore, the health infrastructure is unevenly allocated, with the urban areas found to have a higher concentration of hospitals. Among the surveyed districts, the shortfall in PHCs and CHCs was mostly found in Rohtas and West Champaran. Human resources, like doctors, ANMs, and other staff, were largely short in the Madhubani district. The outbreak of the AES epidemic in 2019 and of the COVID-19 crisis magnified the real picture of the healthcare facilities in the state. The accessibility of the health infrastructure presents an intimidating scenario.

The shortfall in the healthcare resources affects the poor families as they continue to be a major stakeholder of public facilities. The non-availability of the resources not only affects the health outcomes but also increases out-of-pocket expenditure due to the increasing use of private facilities and exacerbates vulnerabilities. The state government is attempting to strengthen the health sector by investing more in the health infrastructure. There was a stimulus increase in per capita public spending from Rs. 330 in 2014–2015 to Rs. 771 in 2019–2020 (Bihar Economic Survey 2019–2020). To make a breakthrough in the poor health system, several social and healthcare programmes have been initiated, but the visible gaps in the healthcare resources indicate a need for drastic policy reforms. The structural inequalities—due to the low socioeconomic conditions, alongside a crippled health system—appear to keep the health outcomes at a low level in the state. In order to have an explicit understanding of the linkages between newborn health outcomes and socioeconomic and health services, a deeper investigation into neonatal health by differentials in socioeconomic attributes is essential. The next section describes the neonatal health situation in the state based on the evidence collected from the field survey.

Newborn Deaths in Bihar: Trends and Differentials

A closer look into the trends in NMR, presented in Fig. 2.1 in Chap. 2 and Fig. 3.1, shows historically neonatal mortality in Bihar is higher than in India. NMR of India has declined gradually over the years, from 32 to 23 per 1000 live births between 2010 and 2018. The newborn mortality in Bihar remains almost stagnant and is higher than the overall NMR of the country. The recently released NFHS-5 phase-1 data reveals a change in the NMR from 36.7 per cent in 2015–2016 to 34.5 per cent in 2019–2020. The SRS figures also reported a 10 per cent decline between 2017 and 2018. The state, however, recorded a higher NMR than the national average and posed a major challenge for the health system of the state. More than three-quarters of infant deaths in the state are neonatal deaths (78.7 per cent), one of the highest, after Odisha (79.4 per cent).

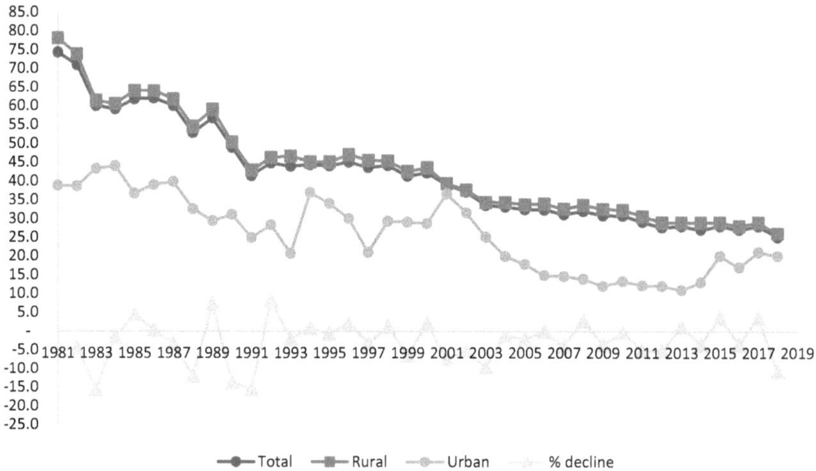

Fig. 3.1 Trends in neonatal mortality in Bihar. (Source: SRS 1981–2018)

The NMR in Bihar was observed to decline by 15.3 per cent during 1990–1991 and by 13 per cent between 2010 and 2011. Following that, there was stagnancy until the state experienced a further dip of 10 per cent in 2017–2018. The rural-urban differential in the NMR shows that the NMR is much higher in rural Bihar than in urban Bihar. However, the NMR in urban Bihar shows an upward trend since 2014. The trends in the NMR show that the factors contributing to neonatal mortality in the state have not been effectively addressed; hence, the pathways that influence NMR are paramount for effective policy interventions.

The survey data collected shows that neonatal deaths stand at 22 per 1000 live births. Among the reported causes of death, prematurity/low birth weight is a major cause (27 per cent), followed by asphyxia (24 per cent). Congenital malfunctions, infections (sepsis/diarrhoea/pneumonia), and jaundice contribute less than 10 per cent. These findings corroborate the findings of other studies that prematurity and low birth weight, birth asphyxia/trauma, and congenital malformations are the leading causes of neonatal deaths (Dandona et al. 2019). Most of the deaths, especially of those born at home, are not medically certified. The cause of death of 30 per cent of the neonates in this study could not be identified and was categorised as unknown causes. That most of the deaths occur in the early neonatal period (Fig. 3.2) is also supported by the

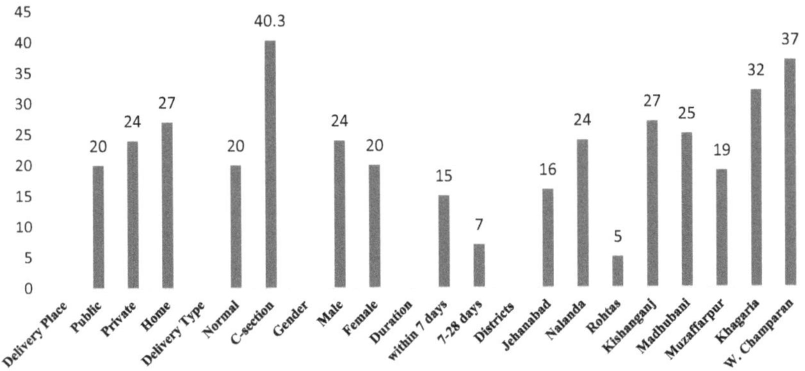

Fig. 3.2 Variations in neonatal deaths by different attributes. (Source: Field data)

existing data. Death within 7 days of birth accounted for 15 deaths per 1000 live births. The figure was reduced by almost half (to 7 per 1000 live births) in the late neonatal period. The findings about neonatal death by type and nature of delivery reiterate the role of institutional care in newborn survival. Women who delivered at home reported a higher neonatal death, primarily because of deliveries conducted by traditional birth attendants and a lack of knowledge about care practices. The socioeconomically backward districts, having poor health infrastructure, such as West Champaran, Khagaria, Kishanganj, and Madhubani, recorded higher neonatal deaths than those of better-off districts.

Not only does Bihar suffer from economic impoverishment, but also is a gender disparate state. Various studies have documented gender differences in infant mortality, pointing out the higher mortality among girls in the post-neonatal period. Contrasts in the pattern of NMR among boys and girls persist in the South Asian countries and many Indian states; gender disadvantages in the early neonatal mortality have been reported in the study area. In our study, although the overall NMR was higher among males (24) than females (20), more deaths were observed among female neonates (17) than the male (15) ones in the early neonatal period. Previous studies in South Asian countries, including India, have shown a lower risk of death among males than females, reflecting disparities in treatment (Alkema et al. 2014). The strong son preference, prevalent in some cultural settings, results in discrimination in healthcare use (Das Gupta 1987) and increases the social risk for girls much more than the biological risk for boys (Arnold et al. 1998; Lawn et al. 2014). These cultural values are deeply embedded in Bihar's society and appear to intensify the familial negligence of care for female newborns, contributing to excess female early neonatal death.

Caesarean delivery has proved to provide survival advantage (Molina et al. 2015); contrary to expectation, NMR in the study area was found to be almost double in the case of C-section deliveries (40.3) compared to vaginal deliveries (20). In India, C-section deliveries increased several folds, from 2.6 per cent in 1992–1993 (NFHS-1) to 21.5 in 2019–2021(NFHS-4). A similar pattern was seen in Bihar, where C-section increased from 6.2 per cent in 2015–2016 to 9.7 per cent in 2019–2020. While caesarean delivery is generally recommended for certain obstetric complications (Hibbered 1976), the privatisation of healthcare has driven the trend of C-section deliveries (Ghosh and James 2010). The existing evidence suggests that C-section without labour complications does not improve neonatal survival but rather increases the risk of neonatal mortality (MacDorman et al. 2008). Besides delivery complications, the lack of birth preparedness may also lead to adverse consequences. These findings highlight the need for an increased focus on care of mother and postnatal care of newborns.

Differentials in Neonatal Deaths by Socio-demographic and Service-Related Attributes

It is well known that utilisation of MNH care and care practices are often linked to deep-rooted social and cultural factors and interact in many ways that are not always clearly understood (WHO 2006). Chapter 2 illustrates that neonatal death is caused by a combination of factors. This section summarises the socioeconomic differentials in the use of healthcare services and its linkages with neonatal deaths to explore the underlying barriers to newborn survival.

The chances of newborn survival were found to be lower for mothers of younger age, those with closely spaced pregnancies, and those having a lack of education. Respondents who had a birth spacing of less than a year had 114 deaths per 1000 live births, which declined steadily for the longer birth intervals of four years and above to 14 per 1000 live births. These results corroborate the findings of other studies that biomedical factors have a significant effect on newborn survival (Titaley et al. 2008). Neonates born in rural areas, in SC/ST or poor families, and to less-educated mothers and those women least exposed to mass media have lower chances of survival. Surprisingly, Hindus experienced more neonatal deaths compared to other religions in the study area. This shows that survival disadvantages being concentrated in the low socioeconomic groups and rural Bihar are attributable to lack of knowledge, adherence to cultural norms, discrimination, and higher cost and lack of supply of services. This also shows that the use of health services is not uni-dimensional and does not increase by a mere improvement in supply and that rather, it is determined by a complex set of factors such as the attitude of people, their knowledge and awareness of the health problems, and the affordability of the services (Simon 2008).

The survey data revealed that a higher level of access to MNH services such as early registration of pregnancy, safe delivery, and visits of ASHA increased the chances of newborn survival. Quality of care—a composite index of availability, affordability, and service delivery—is significant in neonatal health. Women who reported poor QoC experienced more neonate deaths and vice-versa and these findings corroborate the existing evidence on the association of quality of services with newborn survival (Coffey 2019; Ghosh and Dinda 2018). To reach a large target audience, auxiliary nurse midwives (ANMs) set up immunisation and iron-folic acid (IFA) distribution camps in Anganwadi Centres (AWCs), where the mass gathering does not allow time for each pregnant woman to be screened completely for any complications that may be present with the potential to cause neonatal death. Place of uptake of ANC thus is significantly associated with newborn health. Women accessing ANC from AWCs are unable to have their complications addressed due to the lack of facilities. This is why women with pregnancy complications had more deaths (68 per 1000 live births) than those with uncomplicated deliveries (14 per 1000 live births) in the study area. Women who can afford a better quality of care access facilities that can minimise adverse outcomes (Singh et al. 2013). The use of these services, however, is also patterned by socioeconomic inequalities and service-related challenges, which need further exploration.

Summary

The state is on a path of positive transformation; yet sluggishness persists in socioeconomic development and healthcare achievements. Bihar is the poorest state, with socio-demographic indicators so lousy that they drag down all of India's. In response to socioeconomic and health system adversities, Bihar continues to fail to accomplish many of its health targets, including neonatal mortality. In the study area, it was found that the neonatal deaths are disproportionately experienced by the poor, the less-educated, and the marginalised households and MNH service utilisation increases the chances of survival. A manifold increase in facility birth, however, has gone unaccompanied with a comparable improvement in newborn survival, indicating that the policy measures likely did not consider the quality of the services provided. The study provides evidence on the importance of quality of care for newborn survival. This implies that the supply-side constraints should be addressed by focusing on the complex challenges of the health system. A well-functioning health system, with an improved quality of care and equity-based interventions, is recommended to improve neonatal survival in the state. Socioeconomic development and healthcare reforms have undoubtedly altered the orientation of individuals towards a greater use of MNH services. However, there exist inequities in the access to health service utilisation that necessitate exploring the local and cultural factors affecting newborn survival in the state. Understanding the drivers and structural forces that influence the health-seeking behaviour of women and the newborn, therefore, is important to explore barriers that impede the use of newborn health services.

References

All India Survey on Higher Education (AISHE), Ministry of Education, Department of Higher Education, Government of India, New Delhi 2019–2020.

Alkema, L., Chao, F., You, D., Pedersen, J., & Sawyer, C. C. (2014). National, regional, and global sex ratios of infant, child, and under-5 mortality and identification of countries with outlying ratios: a systematic assessment. *The Lancet Global Health*, *2*(9), e521–e530.

Arnold, F., Choe, M. K., & Roy, T. K. (1998). Son preference, the family-building process and child mortality in India. *Population Studies*, *52*(3), 301–315.

Avinash Kumar (2020): COVID-19 and the Public Health System in Bihar, *Economic and Political Weekly*, Vol. 55(16).

Bhattacharya, G. (2009). Intra-state disparity in government expenditure: An analysis. *Economic and Political Weekly*, 231–237.

Bihar Economic Survey (2019–2020). Government of Bihar, Finance Department.

Census (2011) https://censusindia.gov.in/census_and_you/migrations.aspx

Chakravarti, A. (2001). Caste and agrarian class: A view from Bihar. *Economic and Political Weekly*, 1449–1462.
Coffey, D. (2019). The association between neonatal death and facility birth in regions of India. *Demographic Research*, *40*, 417–430.
Dandona, R., Kumar, G. A., Bhattacharya, D., Akbar, M., Atmavilas, Y., Nanda, P., & Dandona, L. (2019). Distinct mortality patterns at 0–2 days versus the remaining neonatal period: results from population-based assessment in the Indian state of Bihar. *BMC Medicine*, *17*(1), 1–19.
Das Gupta, Monica 1987 Selective Discrimination against Female Children in Rural Punjab, India. *Population and Development Review* 13: 77–100.
Diwakar, D.M. & Mehendru, A. (2020) *Mapping growth and inequality in Bihar (an inter-district analysis, in Mapping inequality in Bihar)*. Report prepared by A.N. Sinha Institute of Social Studies & Oxfam India.
Ghosh, D., & Dinda, S. (2018). Health infrastructure and economic development in India. In *Health Economics and Healthcare Reform: Breakthroughs in Research and Practice* (pp. 78–97). IGI Global.
Ghosh, S., & James, K. S. (2010). Levels and trends in caesarean births: cause for concern? *Economic and Political Weekly*, 19–22.
Hibbered, LT (1976). Changing Trends in Caesarean Section, *American Journal of Obstetrics & Gynecology*, 125: 798–804.
Lawn, J. E., Blencowe, H., Oza, S., You, D., Lee, A. C., Waiswa, P., ... Lancet Every Newborn Study Group. (2014). Every Newborn: progress, priorities, and potential beyond survival. *The Lancet*, *384*(9938), 189–205.
MacDorman, M. F., Declercq, E., Menacker, F., & Malloy, M. H. (2008). Neonatal mortality for primary cesarean and vaginal births to low-risk women: Application of an "intention-to-treat" model. *Birth*, *35*(1), 3–8.
Molina, G., Weiser, T. G., Lipsitz, S. R., Esquivel, M. M., Uribe-Leitz, T., Azad, T., ... Haynes, A. B. (2015). Relationship between cesarean delivery rate and maternal and neonatal mortality. *Jama*, *314*(21), 2263–2270.
National Family Health Survey in India, NFHS-5, 2019–2020, IIPS Mumbai.
National Family Health Survey in India, NFHS-3, 2005–2006, IIPS Mumbai.
National Health Profile (2018). Published by Cental Bureau of Health Intelligence, Ministry of Health and Family Welfare.
Periodic Labour Force Survey, Annual Report 2018–2019. Ministry of Statistics and Programme Implementation, National Statistics Office, GoI.
Prasad, P. H., & Rodgers, G. B. (1983). *Class, caste and landholding in the analysis of the rural economy* (No. 1914-2017-2040).
Ranjan, M., & Dwivedi, L. K. (2019). Death clustering in India: Levels, trends, and differentials, 1992–2016. *Indian Journal of Child Health*, *6*(4), 165–172.
Rodgers, Gerry. (2012). *Understanding Unequal Economic and Social Outcomes in Rural Bihar: The Importance of Caste, Class and Landholding*. New Delhi: Institute for Human Development.

Rural Health Statistics, 2019–2020.
Sample Registration System (2018). Office of Registrar General of India, GOI.
Simon, T. (2008, September). Health care accessibility in Kerala: An analysis across different socioeconomic groups. In *5th Annual Conference of the HDCA*, New Delhi, India.
Singh, A., Kumar, A., & Kumar, A. (2013). Determinants of neonatal mortality in rural India, 2007–2008. *PeerJ*, *1*, e75.
Titaley, C. R., Dibley, M. J., Agho, K., Roberts, C. L., & Hall, J. (2008). Determinants of neonatal mortality in Indonesia. *BMC Public Health*, *8*(1), 1–15.
World Bank. (2016). 'Bihar: Poverty, Growth and Inequality'. World Bank. Retrieved February 20, 2020, from http://documents.worldbank.org/curated/en/781181467989480762/pdf/105842-BRI-P157572-PUBLIC-Bihar-Poverty.pdf
World Health Organization. (2006). Neonatal and perinatal mortality: country, regional and global estimates. World Health Organization. https://apps.who.int/iris/handle/10665/43444

CHAPTER 4

Access Barriers to Antenatal Care and Facility Delivery

Introduction

A mother and her newborn have undeniable healthcare needs, and there is a consensus that the continuum of care from pregnancy to the neonatal period is key to improving MNH outcomes (Coffey 2019). The ICPD conference (1994) of 173 countries including India recommended reproductive health as a basic human right and a priority for global health. The National Population Policy (2000) reiterated India's commitment to safe motherhood programmes and emphasised the promotion of MNCH services as an important component of family welfare programmes. But access to maternal, newborn, and child healthcare services depends on the ability to obtain these services (Rutaremwa et al. 2015). To reinforce the health system and curb the menace of maternal and child mortality, the National Rural Health Mission was launched in 2005. Despite all the efforts, almost half of the pregnant women do not complete four ANC visits, and only one-fifth have access to full ANC. Institutional delivery has increased manifold, especially in the public sector. However, a significant variation persists across states and socioeconomic groups.

Utilisation of MNH services is a challenge in low-income countries, particularly in sub-Saharan Africa and South Asia. By 2019, while over three-quarters (62 per cent) of women received antenatal care (UNICEF 2019) globally, in India, the figure was less than half, with a wide regional inequality. As per the National Family Health Survey (NFHS) data

S. R. Mahapatro, *Towards Newborn Survival*,
https://doi.org/10.1007/978-981-19-3417-9_4

(2015–2016), full ANC is unacceptably low (3.3 per cent) and only 14 per cent received minimum four ANC in Bihar. The NFHS-5 data reveals a further increase in ANC and delivery care in the state, with a quarter of all women having accessed four ANC, and three-quarters having had an institutional delivery. Although there is a visible improvement in the use of MNH services, the status of service utilisation is comparatively lower than in many other poor-performing states and national average. This raises the question as to whether the ongoing health interventions and policies take into account the underlying adversities that impede the use of newborn health services. Given the complex socioeconomic structure, a large population base, and persistent traditional cultural practices, uncovering the barriers to utilising maternal and newborn healthcare in the state warrants further investigation.

Studies that have analysed maternal and newborn health care in low-income settings have found cultural attitudes, poverty, and lack of education, together with a poor healthcare system, to be the major impediments to ameliorating maternal and newborn health. However, systematic variations in the determinants have been observed in different socioeconomic and cultural contexts. For instance, a study by Navaneetham and Dharmalingam (2002) on the determinants of ANC in the South Indian states found that education and wealth status were significant predictors in Karnataka; caste was significant in Andhra Pradesh but not in Karnataka. In this regard, Basu (1990) revealed that the success of health interventions relies on the ability to confirm people's lifestyle, which requires a prior knowledge of the health culture of the population. Thus, demographic and socioeconomic determinants alone are not sufficient to account for the use of MNH services. Community norms and beliefs, mediated through these social determinants, shape the perceived benefits and risks of using the health services. In conjunction with the demand-side attributes, the health system structure and functioning also have a prominence in influencing the utilisation of MNH services.

The present chapter discusses two components of maternal and newborn health—access to antenatal care and choice of place of delivery—based on the field data collected. Section two clarifies the status of and differentials in utilisation of antenatal healthcare. Section three is on the choice of place of delivery and its differentials. The barriers to the use of ANC and institution for delivery are discussed in the last section of the chapter.

Status of and Differentials in Antenatal Service Utilisation

The antenatal period is a window of opportunity for identifying and preventing pregnancy complications and hence, adverse birth outcomes (Chauhan 2012; Singh et al. 2014a). The ANC visits provide an opportunity to access quality of care—consummation of IFA, immunisation against tetanus, screening of and treatment of diseases, and strengthening of contact between healthcare providers and pregnant women. Bulk of the studies in developing countries shows that increasing utilisation of ANC reduces preterm delivery, prevents birth asphyxia, and increases the weight of neonates (Zeng et al. 2008), and there is chances of successful transition from pregnancy to labour and delivery, improves birth outcomes, and enhances knowledge of postnatal care (Berhan and Berhan 2014).

Consistent with the other studies, the present study too found access to ANC to be a driving force for delivering at a facility and newborn survival. More than half of all neonatal deaths (59 per cent) in the study were among women who had less than three ANC visits. Among mothers who had home deliveries, 27 per cent did not utilise ANC, while among those who delivered at an institution, this figure was as low as 10 per cent. This supports the evidence that ANC visits encourage pregnant women to choose a health facility for delivery as it strengthens the trust relations and enhances the knowledge about the benefits of facility care.

Although the state guarantees free antenatal services, utilisation of MNH services, especially the uptake of full ANC (FANC[1]), is one of the lowest in Bihar (15 per cent only). Despite a universal registration of pregnancy (96 per cent), a significant variation is observed in the uptake of antenatal services (Table 4.1). Nearly 14 per cent respondents went through pregnancy without antenatal care, and a significant drop in the figures from 86 per cent for one visit to 20 per cent for four visits. IFA supplementation, in accordance with the prescribed guidelines, was followed by half of the respondents, whereas TT injections were received by as many as 85 per cent of the respondents. Inter-district variance in the uptake of antenatal services was observed, with Muzaffarpur and Rohtas showing more utilisation and Kishanganj ranking at the bottom. A low

[1] Full ANC in this book follows the NFHS definition: Women who had at least four ANC visits, had taken at least one TT injection/syrup, and consumed IFA tablets for at least 100 days.

Table 4.1 Status of and differentials in ANC utilisation across selected districts

District	*Pregnancy registered*	*Received MCP card*	*At-least one visit*	*Minimum four ANC visits*	*100 IFA*	*2TT*	*Full ANC*	*Did not avail ANC*	*No test*	*N*
Jehanabad	93.9	90.5	86.6	21.5	71.1	85.1	17.5	13.4	1.9	288
Nalanda	95.6	86.7	77.8	17.4	54	75.5	12.9	22.1	1.8	277
Rohtas	97.7	94.1	87.7	21.5	72.6	86.1	19.2	12.3	4.9	296
Kishanganj	91.9	95	80.8	10.9	54.8	79.5	7.1	19.2	12.8	318
Madhubani	96.3	89.5	88.7	19.2	55.3	87.6	14.2	11.2	14.6	319
Muzaffarpur	95.6	86.3	87.5	26.4	51.2	87	19.2	12.4	7.1	294
Khagaria	99.9	95.3	96.8	24.6	57.4	94.9	18.2	3.2	27.5	286
West Champaran	97.4	90.4	89.8	28.1	52.8	87.7	18.2	10.2	6.5	306
Total	**95.5**	**90.1**	**86.1**	**20.2**	**55.2**	**84.8**	**14.7**	**13.9**	**1.6**	**2384**

Source: Field data

level of socioeconomic development in interaction with other contextual factors obstructs the utilisation of ANC in the low-ranking districts. Apart from the comprehensive ANC visits, WHO recommended maternal and foetal screening such as HIV/AIDS test, anaemia and blood pressure check-up, ultra-sound, weight measurement, and so on, as it influences pregnancy outcomes. Of the ANC service recipients, 11 per cent did not undergo any test. The proportion was substantially higher in Khagaria (27.5 per cent), but lower (2 per cent) in Nalanda and Jehanabad. Approximately half of the respondents did not undergo other tests, including HIV/Blood/HB tests, although blood pressure checks and weight measurements and ultra-sound were done by majority. The observation that a significant proportion of women had not undergone many of the essential tests during pregnancy is a matter of concern and calls for rethinking antenatal care policy interventions. The analysis shows little coverage of full ANC across the districts, with much little utilisation in Kishanganj.

Socioeconomic Differentials Among ANC Service Recipients

This section of the chapter presents the socioeconomic differentials in the utilisation of antenatal care and facility delivery (Table 4.2). Education of women and their involvement in household decisions were found to be enablers of ANC utilisation. In the study, women having a higher level of education were found to have availed ANC twice as much as illiterate women. Greater awareness and knowledge of modern healthcare services, improved communication skills, and capability to decide on the use of healthcare services (Caldwell 1979; Chopra et al. 2018) among the educated increase service utilisation. Women empowerment although has a positive influence on access to ANC, full ANC was lower among women who participated in household decision-making. Perhaps working women despite being empowered were not able to get time to access ANC as desired. On the contrary, mass media exposure (watching television and reading newspapers) had a positive effect on the use of full ANC and lessened the discontinuation of services.

The ubiquity of caste-class differences reveals that FANC was disproportionately lower among the poor and the marginalised. While 17 per cent of the upper-caste women received FANC, it was only 12 per cent for the SC/ST. Hindus availed FANC more (15 per cent) than the others (13 per cent). Muslim women had less autonomy and interacted less with the

Table 4.2 Distribution of respondents according to access to ANC and place of delivery by socio-demographic characteristics and facilitating factors

		Antenatal care			*Place of delivery*			
Socioeconomic factors		*Discontinued*	*Full ANC*	*p-value*	*Health facility*	*Home/others*	*p-value*	*N*
Current age				P<0.001			P<0.001	
15–19	12.2	74.3	13.5		84.5	15.5		175
20–24	10	74.7	15.3		80.6	19.4		1011
25–29	16.6	66.3	17.1		74.9	25		822
30 & above	19	72.8	8.2		73.8	26.2		376
Children ever born				P<0.001			P<0.001	
1 to 2	11.6	71.7	16.7		82.2	17.9		1385
3 to 4	15.9	71.2	12.9		74.2	25.8		774
5 & above	22.4	69.7	7.9		64.5	35.6		225
Level of education				P<0.000			P<0.001	
Illiterate	19	71.6	9.4		69.9	30.1		935
Primary	13.7	72.7	13.6		78.7	21.3		737
Secondary	7	70.9	22.1		87.8	12.2		327
Higher secondary & above	7.2	68.2	24.6		88.7	11.3		385
Caste				p<0.005			P<0.001	
SC/ST	16.8	70.9	12.3		74.6	25.4		240
OBC	12.6	71.9	15.5		79.9	20.1		1298
General	12.2	70.1	17.7		77.7	22.4		846
empowerment				P<0.045				
No	14.2	70.6	15.2		79.2	20.8		2085
Yes	12.7	76.4	10.9		78.2	21.8		299
Economic status				p<0.000			P<0.001	
Lowest	18.9	71.7	9.4		71	29		483
Lower	15.2	72.9	11.9		78	22		496

Middle	15	73.5	11.5		79.7	20.3		463
Rich	11.9	68.6	19.5		80	20		479
Richest	9.4	70.1	20.5		79.7	20.3		463
Ever worked				p = 0.402			P<0.001	
No	13.9	71.3	14.8		30.1	69.7		2157
Yes	19.6	68.6	11.8		69.8	30.3		227
Facilitating factors								
Did not receive ANC					10.2	26.9		332
Received full ANC					16.7	7.1		353
Not aware of ANC					7.8	21.8		255
Did not receive MCP card	22.1 332	7.54 1697	9.01 355		8.5	14.9		235
Received ANC from AWC	–	96.8	3.2	322	15.4	30.4		345
ASHA suggested on MNCH care	26.5(330)	57(1697)	62(355)		55.4	45.9		1273
Not suggested by ASHA for facility delivery	–	–	–		3.7	5.7		55
Community-level participation	13.2(330)	17.9(1697)	21(355)		80	20		1881

Source: Field data

outside world and, hence, were less informed about modern healthcare services. While examining the impact of caste/religion, studies show that whereas the under-utilisation of maternal healthcare services among SC/ST women is a result of spatial disadvantages, combined with socioeconomic seclusion, in the case of religious groups, it's the differences in cultural practices and beliefs that result in the variations in the use of maternal care (Navaneetham and Dharmalingam 2002). A clear class gradient was observed where ANC utilisation among the poor was more than two times lower than the richest. Financial difficulties and lack of health information could be the probable reasons among the poor in accessing less ANC services (Singh et al. 2014b).

The influence of demographic factors, such as late age of childbearing and higher parity, lowers the utilisation of ANC. In India's socio-cultural fabric, women must visit their natal home for delivery, specifically during their first pregnancy. Proper communication and lack of hesitation with parents about their health and pregnancy lead their families to take appropriate care, giving adequate attention and, hence, increasing the utilisation of ANC. The confidence gained from the experience of the first birth and the higher age at subsequent births reduces their inclination to use ANC for the higher birth order (Bhatia and Cleland 1995). That said, the study also found that many women were reluctant to consume IFA tablets due to the fear of side effects, which also served to discourage them from having ANC check-ups. A rural-urban gap in utilisation of ANC was observed with higher use among urban than rural women. The diffusion of modern healthcare and the exposure to the modern culture in urban areas increase access to ANC; however no significant differentials in ANC discontinuation by the socioeconomic attributes had been observed except education, whereby illiterate women reported more discontinuation.

The availability and quality of health services were found to have an impact on the use of ANC. Women's participation in the community and interaction with the health workers increased their use of ANC. The survey found that the discontinuation rate was higher among women who opted from Anganwadi Centres (96.8 per cent) and public facilities (84.5 per cent) than the ones who visited private facilities (76.1 per cent). While commenting on the quality of ANC, almost 10 per cent respondents who had received ANC from public providers reported of being dissatisfied with the quality, only 3.2 per cent received full ANC from AWC. The figure increased to 15.6 per cent in the case of public facilities and to 24 per cent in the case of private ones.

Choice of Place of Delivery: Home Versus Institutions

As evidenced by safe motherhood studies, in low- and middle-income countries, place of delivery often determines the quality of care received and, hence, neonatal mortality. An increase in neonatal resuscitation, accompanied by an increase in facility birth, medically corrected birth assistance, and a sanitary environment, leads to more chances of newborn survival (Goudar et al. 2015; Altman et al. 2017).

Despite an unprecedented increase in facility birth, Bihar continues to record comparatively more home deliveries as compared to other states in India. Newborn death is higher for home deliveries (27 per 1000 live births) which is 24 and 20 per 1000 live birth in private and public facilities respectively. This has clearly brought out the importance of institutional care for newborn survival. Unidentified high-risk pregnancies, absence of skilled birth attendance, and lack of knowledge on postnatal care practices reduce the chances of survival of newborns delivered at home. The field observations reveal that like ANC, choice of delivery place is also patterned by the socioeconomic attributes of women. In the study area, economic distress, low social status of family, low level of education, experiences from earlier deliveries, and multiparity were factors that led women to deliver at home (Table 4.2).

The investigation into the role of the health system factors in deciding the place of delivery revealed that interaction with health workers, antenatal visits, and participation in community outreach activities had impacted positively to use institutions. Utilisation of FANC and awareness related to value of services was lower in the case of home delivery (7 per cent) than facility delivery (22 per cent). One in ten respondents who had a facility delivery forewent ANC, while in the case of home delivery, the corresponding figure was almost 27 per cent. Utilisation of MNH services suggested by an ASHA worker was higher among institutional (55 per cent) than home deliveries (45 per cent). Women's community participation increased their health-seeking behaviour as almost 80 per cent of those who did so delivered in a facility. This indicates that health interventions, designed keeping in mind communication linkages of the health workers with the target population, facilitate the use of reproductive and newborn health services.

To unearth the factors behind the choice of place of delivery, the respondents were asked to elucidate the reasons for their choice. Almost three-quarters of the respondents delivered at home mainly due to the sudden labour pain combined with a delay in making a decision (17 per cent) and lack of transportation to reach a facility (25 per cent). Another factor that prohibited women from visiting a facility for delivery was the role of the family in decision-making (35 per cent). The patriarchal nature of the family and resistance by older women led them to go for home delivery. While a few studies have emphasised on the demand-side barriers like unwillingness of family members, misreporting of labour pains (Gorain et al. 2017), and fear of hospital as the major reasons for home delivery, others have pointed out distance to the facility and cost of services as factors discouraging facility delivery (Devasenapathy et al. 2014). In the study more than 10 per cent of the respondents reported distance to the facility and lack of social support as the reasons.

Home delivery is a community practice established firmly in low socio-cultural settings. The belief that delivery is a natural process not requiring medical attention is particularly strong in North Bihar. Community practice as the reason behind home delivery was reported by 3.5 per cent of the respondents and it is higher in the Rohtas district (around one-fifth of the home delivery). As the district has a substantial share of tribal population, norms and beliefs of such community influence the choice of place of delivery. Safe delivery and monetary incentive were the most preferred reasons for facility delivery in the survey area, and pregnancy complications stood out as a striking reason for opting for private over public facilities. Around 13 per cent of the women reported complications, and it was almost five times higher in the case of delivery in private facilities compared to the public ones. This difference possibly arises as most public health institutions have a limited infrastructure and limited manpower and are under-equipped due to which they make last-minute referrals to private hospitals.

More than three-fourths of the respondents had opted for institutional delivery in the survey districts, with a higher proportion in public facilities (58 per cent) than private facilities (20 per cent). Home deliveries attended by SBAs were too few in the surveyed districts (4.5 per cent). A skewed pattern in the choice of place of delivery was observed, with districts located in the southern region—the socioeconomically developed ones reporting fewer home deliveries than the north. Access to MNH services, thus, is the reflection of the socio-cultural context and availability of health services.

Barriers to Institutional Care: ANC Services and Facility Delivery

Many vertical programmes have been implemented under NHM as part of the safe motherhood intervention to overcome the challenges of utilisation of MNCH services. These programmes include the Reproductive, Maternal, Newborn, Child, and Adolescent Health (RMNCH+A) Strategy, Direct Benefit Transfer, community-based interventions, and so on. Health workers were recruited on a large scale under NRHM for counselling and mobilising pregnant women through behavioural change interventions and upscaling the use of MNH service. Despite the expansion and provision of free facility care, many pregnant women are deprived of access to quality services. This suggests the barriers to utilisation of MNH care have not been addressed adequately by the healthcare interventions. Studies across the globe show that the utilisation of MNH services is conditioned by demand- and supply-side factors and linked to cultural norms, socioeconomic conditions, perceptions of clients and community, affordability of services, and supply of quality services (Leone et al. 2013).

Demand-Side Barriers

This section presents evidences on the underlying demand-side mechanisms related to personal, household, and community attributes that pattern the utilisation of antenatal services and choice of place of delivery.

Socioeconomic Inequality and Use of MNH Services

Health inequity is a serious public health concern and addressing it is central to achieving health-related SDGs. The implementation of pro-poor maternal and child health programmes in the state has resulted in an incremental change in the utilisation of MNH services but unequally, with a considerable barrier to much of the population maintained and class-caste inequalities play an important role in this regard.

In the Indian society, the underprivileged fall outside the sphere of MNCH interventions and are deprived of basic facilities due to social discrimination, exclusion, and economic challenges. The class differences in healthcare utilisation are mainly attributable to the lower capacity to pay by the poor. Having poor economic and marginalised status, this section of women was more deprived in terms of availing the recommended number of antenatal visits and having institutional delivery. While lack of awareness was a major cause behind the non-use of services, it was higher among scheduled castes/tribes (13.5 per cent) than other social classes (9 per cent). The traditional community practices prevailed more among the low caste groups, which persuaded them to depend on the informal modes of delivery and child care practices. Almost 10 per cent of the SC/ST women who had delivered in a health facility reported that the medical staff's behaviour was not appropriate; the corresponding figure among the upper-caste women was around 5 per cent. These evidences reflect that discrimination and provider's bias towards the lower castes still prevail in the various delivery points, which reduces the motivation to access healthcare.

Similar to studies by Skordis-Worrall et al. (2011), the study shows the delivery of services is inequitably distributed and favoured the better-off section to a larger extent. It is estimated that OOPE on delivery among the poorest was 1.12 times higher than the total household budget which was 0.53 times among the richest. Many a times the poor had to go for distress financing to meet the delivery and newborn health expenditure. Higher burden of out-of-pocket expenditure (OOPE) and economic distress not only discourages the poor from accessing healthcare, but the neighbourhood effect on utilising MNCH services also becomes negative and resulted in poor health outcomes.

Role of Gender and Intra-household Decision-Making

Intra-familial decision-making power is a strong predictor of the choice of place of delivery in low-income regions. In rural areas, the young adolescents are unable to ascertain their determination to seek maternal and child healthcare owing to their lower decision-making power. In the socio-cultural context of Bihar, the decision as to the place of delivery is not the prerogative of the women alone. The patriarchal norms and gender inequalities that prevail in the cultural context of Bihar lower the bargaining power of the women in household decisions, including those pertaining to their own health. In the study area, the decision regarding the place of delivery was mainly shaped by the voices of husband and elderly members, especially mother-in-law. Only one in four respondents made their own decision about the place of delivery and decisions were reported to be made jointly. A majority of three-quarter of women who had the autonomy in household decisions and delivered in a health facility reveals the choice of place of delivery is undermined by the status of women in the family.

More than half respondents who delivered at home preferred having an institutional delivery, which they could not do. Alongside low status, lack of knowledge about the onset of labour and delay in the decision to access care were the underlying reasons. The three-delay model, that comprises delay in decision, delay in reaching a facility, and delayed care, affects the pregnancy outcomes. In Bihar, the first delay, that is, delay in decision to avail care is particularly challenging. The absence of the husband due to migration impacts the healthcare utilisation among pregnant women. Men having the knowledge of pregnancy, childbirth, and postpartum complications were more likely to have all maternal health services utilised by their wives (Jungari and Paswan 2019). Among the home deliveries, the husbands of 19 per cent respondents were away at the time of the delivery. Lower use of antenatal care, disinclination of family for facility delivery, and lower visits of ASHA were comparatively more prevalent in migrant households. Almost three-fifths of the migrant wives thought that husband's absence had an impact on the decision regarding the place of delivery.

Tradition and Culture

At the root of the low uptake of health services in the state are unquestioning cultural beliefs and social norms. The cultural beliefs of the community are reflected in an individual's health decisions because their behaviour is influenced by how the community views their actions. In Bihar, like in many places in South Asian countries, the tradition of early marriage, the culture of son preference, and the practice of early childbearing are widely prevalent, revealing many facts about the health and social position of women. Younger maternal age at conception was very common in the study area as almost three among four women aged 15–19 had delivered their first child. For these young women who had entered the institution of marriage, childbearing soon after marriage was a social norm, a symbol of marriage, and that established their social status within the family. In such a society, girls do not exhibit any agency in marriage. Further, lack of knowledge on the family planning measures and in many instances use of any birth control method which is considered as a social taboo restricts the use of family planning measures and hence, women become pregnant easily.

In the study area, the uptake of full ANC was lower in the late age as also in the young age. Pregnant women of late age and higher parity showed reluctance for institutional delivery. The perceived difficulties of institutional birth due to their own previous experience and experience of giving birth safely at home or that of other women of the community made them refrain from visiting a facility.

One of the respondents who had a home delivery reported:

> *I did not avail ANC due to the fear of injection. My mother-in-law said home delivery is better than hospital delivery. My husband was absent at that time. Had he been present, I might have decided to go to the hospital.* (Sangeeta Devi, Age 25, Madhubani)

Another respondent reported:

> *Since I was in good health, there was no need to go to the hospital for a check-up. The cash incentive was also not sufficient enough to cover the cost of delivery, nor receiving it in a timely manner. So it was good to deliver at home.* (Manju, Age 30, Nalanda District)

Health Behaviour: Preference Versus Perception

The health behaviour of people is closely linked to the socio-cultural environment of the community they are living in. The belief in the traditional methods embedded in the many cultural settings of the study area had a strong influence on the choice of place of delivery. The community beliefs or norms intercede through household and individual factors influence the perceptions about health service utilisation (Kifle et al. 2018). Home is the preferred place stated by around 30 per cent of the mothers who delivered at home. Those women explained the comfort of delivering at home from earlier experience (35 per cent) with no fear of undergoing a C-section (33 per cent), motivated them to opt for a home delivery. Further there was a belief that TBAs/dais are connoisseurs and that they can conduct a delivery much more safely. In the survey we had asked respondents of home delivery about their perception regarding skill of TBA, and 44 per cent had the perception that TBAs and doctors had the same level of skill, and around 5 per cent stated that TBAs were more skilled than the doctors.

Among the perceived barriers to institutional delivery, the high cost of care was reported by more than half of the respondents (52 per cent). Lack of trust (29 per cent) and negative approach of service providers (24 per cent) were the next two most commonly reported reasons.

> *We have no trust in facility care. My mother-in-law said that she had taken her daughter to the hospital for delivering the baby. However, given the kind of treatment my family received, we lost trust in facility delivery. So my mother-in-law refused to take me to the hospital despite the ASHA workers suggesting so.* (Fulo Devi, Age 25, Rohtas District)

One respondent, who did not receive ANC and had a home delivery, said:

> *Even though I was aware of ANC services, due to the fear of receiving the injection, I did not go to the facility.*

System-Level Barriers

The system-level barriers are related to the efficacy of service delivery and cost of healthcare services.

Community-Level Interactions and Service Utilisation

In resource-constrained settings, community-level interventions facilitate service utilisation to a larger extent. By enhancing awareness, transforming social beliefs, and improving interpersonal communication, such initiatives improve the use of MNCH services. Community health workers (CHWs) are the social and cultural intermediaries strengthening the interface between the existing health system and the community (Lehmann et al. 2004) and play a critical role in addressing the social-cultural barriers towards the utilisation of MNH services. The significance of CHWs became prominent with the Alma Ata Declaration in 1978. For this, frontline workers are trained and incentivised under NRHM to raise awareness about healthcare services through community-level meetings or home visits. In resource-poor settings, midwife-led continuity of care reduces preterm births by up to 24 per cent (WHO 2020) and this finding of this study is also supported this.

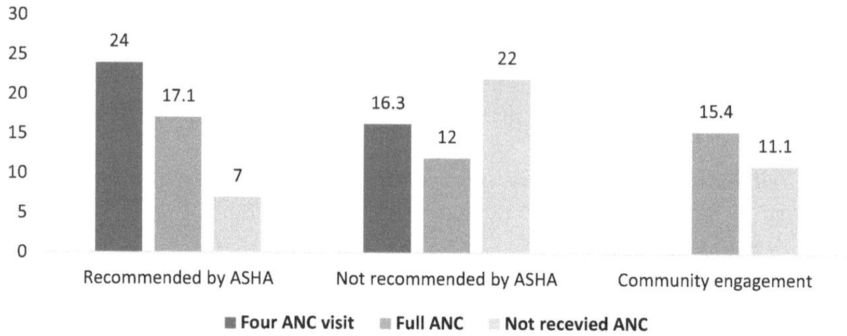

Fig. 4.1 Community-level interventions and ANC utilisation. (Source: Field data)

Fig. 4.1 shows that ASHA as a facilitator increases the uptake of four ANC visits. Of those who had not availed ANC, 22 per cent had not received any suggestions from ASHA, whereas 7 per cent did receive suggestions but did not act on them. The propensity to have four or more visits was higher among women who had received the advice of an ASHA worker (24 per cent) than those who had not (16.3 per cent). A similar association could be observed with full antenatal check-up. Among the women who visited an AWC, nearly three-fifths did not receive any recommendation by ASHA workers on maternal and childcare practices during pregnancy. Similarly, around 30 per cent of women who discontinued ANC from a public facility reported not having been informed by an ASHA worker. The figure shows that the participation of women in community outreach services improved their chances of ANC uptake (15.4 per cent for participation vs. 11.1 per cent for non-participation).

ANC visits facilitate women's access to institutional care as the interactions with health workers during ANC visit develop trust relations and provide opportunity to assess the quality of the services. The association of place of delivery and community engagement provided the evidence that most of the women who delivered at a facility had participated in the community (Table 4.2). The community workers played a positive role in changing the family perception of facility delivery. Almost three in five women delivered in public facility received recommendation by an ASHA worker. These facts reveal positive role of ASHA workers in upscaling utilisation of MNH services.

The study, however, found that the coverage of eligible women by the frontline workers was not universal. Almost half of them (47 per cent) were not informed about antenatal services, and the proportion was higher among the non-utilisers (74 per cent). This was further supported by the evidence on medicines/supplements recommended during the visit. Around one-fifth of the respondents (23 per cent) were not recommended to take IFA tablets. Only 25 per cent were advised to take a Vitamin A supplement, and only 13 per cent were advised to take calcium. While identifying the reasons for the low coverage, it was observed that the service providers also faced certain challenges like lack of adequate compensation. Many times, being overworked de-motivated them and, at other times, their personality traits—such as their communication skills, their ability to reach out to the community, or their prejudice towards a certain community—restricted the participation of the pregnant women.

During the fieldwork, Renu Bala, an ASHA worker from the Muzaffarpur district, said in an interview:

> *Women, especially Muslims, are reluctant to visit a facility. As per the cultural norms, a few months into the pregnancy, women general move to their natal homes for delivery, particularly for the first child, and we are not able to track them.*

She added that they had not got any incentive for a long time from the health department for the service they had delivered. This was demotivating them from continuing to participate in the programme.

Influence of Distance

Lack of geographical access, coupled with inadequate transportation facilities, is the non-monetary barrier to facility-based care and newborn survival (Nesbitt et al. 2016). In rural India, it is seen that each additional kilometre to the health facility is associated with a 4.4 per cent decline in the probability of facility birth (Kumar et al. 2014). These findings are mirrored in the present book as well.

In the survey, around 9 per cent of the respondents, who did not avail ANC, reported distance as a reason, while 12 per cent respondents who had a home delivery attributed their decision to geographical barriers. Within five kilometres of range from facility, 13 per cent deliveries were at home and the figure increased to 28 per cent for more than five kilometres of distance. The distribution of the respondents who delivered at a facility revealed that 42 per cent deliveries took place at institutions located within five kilometres. The proportion declined significantly and linearly to 30 per cent, 17 per cent, and 11 per cent for 0 km–5 km, 10–15 km, and 15 km and above distance respectively and the association is stronger for marginalised and illiterate women. The locational disadvantages were more pronounced among the low social class; hence mothers from the disadvantaged groups should be facilitated more to overcome distance as a constraint to facility delivery.

Cost of Services and Inequality in Health Spending

That maternity cost is a major restraint to the utilisation of institutional care has been recognised widely. Although, theoretically, hospital delivery is free of charge, there are several direct and indirect costs, such as transportation cost, stay, food expenditure, and user fee, that strongly influence women's motivation for choosing the place of delivery. The survey data show around 8 per cent respondents reported high cost of services as the reason for the non-utilisation of institutional care. Among the perceived difficulties of institutional delivery, high cost of service was cited by more than half of the respondents. Estimation shows that one in four mothers resorted to borrowing or selling to meet OOPE (Mishra and Mohanty 2019) and that the extent of distress financing was higher in the poor socioeconomic strata of the low-income states of Bihar and Odisha.

The significant correlation between the use of maternity care and expenditure, evident from the study, suggests that affordability is a major factor determining the use of services. As against the common perception that home delivery would be a minimal cost, we found on an average Rs. 1807/- spent for delivering at home, followed by Rs. 2441 incurred on a delivery in a public health facility. The expenditure was the highest in case of private facilities. The OOPE on delivery in a public facility was Rs. 1509 for those who availed monetary benefits given as part of various cash transfer programmes, whereas it was Rs. 2619 for those who had not registered for any maternity benefit programme reflects the positive role of financial interventions. However, the cost associated with the uptake of ANC and delivery at a facility was higher than the subsidy provided by any programme. Irrespective of the services used, medicines and diagnosis expenditure comprised major expenditure. In the study it consists more than three-fourths of the total ANC expenditure, medicine expenditure alone constituted almost 42 per cent of the total delivery expenditure. Transportation cost and doctor/staff fee constituted 18 per cent and 20

Table 4.3 Expenditure on ANC and delivery care

Item	*ANC services*		*Place of delivery*		
	Public	*Private*	*Public*	*Private*	*Home*
Doctor/staff fee	252	766	586	11,105	477
Medicine cost	1156	3353	1048	5091	776
Diagnostic cost	855	2152	3	1432	73
Transportation cost	292	2628	439	1138	42
Other	257	2679	245	653	438
Expenditure	2513	6900	2441	19,419	1807
OOPE			**1509**		

Source: Field data

a The expenses here report the total expenses made and do not include the JBSY benefit. Total OOPE upon receiving JBSY was Rs. 1509 (discussed in detail in Chap. 8)

per cent of the delivery expenditure in public facilities, although delivering in such facilities is supposed to be free (Table 4.3).

A major share of the expenditure incurred in a private facility was made up of the doctor's fee, which also included charges for stay in the hospital. Expenditure on medicines was almost five times higher in private than public facilities. Contrary to the common belief, OOPE on delivering at a facility was lower than the cost of a home delivery. The higher cost at home was because of the many material things a family had to pay to the TBA for conducting delivery, like agricultural produce and saree, along with money.

A respondent who had a home delivery commented:

> *Poor quality of care and higher delivery expenditure discouraged us from visiting a facility. Although the government subsidizes the expenditure through cash incentives, one still has to pay a lot of money at the hospital.* (Fulo Devi, Rohtas)

Another respondent reported:

> *We are aware of the cash transfer programme of the government, but we had no money at that time to have a facility delivery. My husband was also absent; hence it was unthinkable to visit a facility for delivery.* (Sangeeta Devi, Jehanabad)

The class differences in delivery expenses in the study showed a linear relation but regressive nature as the lower class spent a higher budget share than the richest class. This made poorer households impoverished and discouraged to avail healthcare and the benefits of JBSY. More than 30 per cent respondents reported they had to borrow money or sell assets for meeting the delivery expenses. Dependency on informal institutions such as moneylenders usually charge a higher rate of interest, and such distress financing pushes households into the poverty trap. These difficulties should be taken into consideration during the planning and implementation of health protection measures in future to ensure universal coverage.

Quality of Care at Institutions

Poor quality of care was found to be an important barrier to newborn survival and service utilisation observed in the study. The utilisation of institutional delivery although commendable in the state, the accompanying improvement in neonatal health outcomes is not impressive. The experiences women have at a facility influence the others in the community to utilise services.

Excerpts from an in-depth interview with a respondent who had made an informed decision to have a home delivery:

> *My husband was absent during the delivery. Even if he were present, I would have given birth at home only. Our family has an aversion to public hospitals since the treatment is not done nicely there. I have given birth to five children. Of them, the baby that I delivered in a public hospital died. The ones who were born at home are all alive. ASHA comes only when it is time to visit the AWC for injections. She does not encourage availing ANC services.*

Discussion

This chapter contributes to understanding the barriers linked to the utilisation of antenatal care and institutional delivery in Bihar. Given the complexity of environment women live in, the under-utilisation of MNH services is not alone attributable to health system constraints. The underlying causes also lie outside the domain of health sector and attributed to the societal and behavioural factors. The maternal and newborn health care needs are deeply rooted in the social matrix. In many instances, the societal norms interacting with the personal and household attributes shape the perception about institutional delivery. The community-level interventions do play important role in behavioural transformation towards access to newborn services. To improve service utilisation and newborn survival, appropriate strategies need to be formulated to reduce the cost of services mainly the medicine cost especially among the poor. Along with the promotion of institutional deliveries, in situations where home deliveries are the only available option, safe home-based delivery and newborn care practices should be extensively promoted.

The preceding analysis presented reveals the quality of services at institutions was an important determinant of newborn survival and endorses further service utilisation. A critical understanding of the quality of services is thus important and is presented in the next chapter. These findings facilitate identification of the priorities and strategies required to improve newborn health and hasten the mortality decline in Bihar.

References

Altman, R., Sidney, K., De Costa, A., Vora, K., & Salazar, M. (2017). Is institutional delivery protective against neonatal mortality among poor or tribal women? A cohort study from Gujarat, India. *Maternal and Child Health Journal*, *21*(5), 1065–1072.

Basu, A. M. (1990). Cultural influences on health care use: two regional groups in India. *Studies in Family Planning*, *21*(5), 275–286.

Berhan, Y., & Berhan, A. (2014). Antenatal care as a means of increasing birth in the health facility and reducing maternal mortality: a systematic review. *Ethiopian Journal of Health Sciences*, *24*, 93–104.

Bhatia, J. C., & Cleland, J. (1995). Determinants of maternal care in a region of South India. *Health Transition Review*, 127–142.

Caldwell, J. C. (1979). Education as a factor in mortality decline an examination of Nigerian data. *Population Studies*, 395–413.

Chauhan, A. (2012). Antenatal care among currently married women in Rajasthan, India. *Asian Pacific Journal of Tropical Disease*, *2*, S617–S623.

Chopra, I., Juneja, S. K., & Sharma, S. (2018). Effect of maternal education on antenatal care utilization, maternal and perinatal outcome in a tertiary care hospital. *Int J Reprod Contraception, Obstet Gynecol*, *8*(1), 247.

Coffey, D. (2019). The association between neonatal death and facility birth in regions of India. *Demographic Research*, *40*, 417–430.

Devasenapathy, N., George, M. S., Jerath, S. G., Singh, A., Negandhi, H., Alagh, G &Zodpey, S. (2014). Why women choose to give birth at home: a situational analysis from urban slums of Delhi. *BMJ Open*, 4(5).

Gorain, A., Barik, A., Chowdhury, A., & Rai, R. K. (2017). Preference in place of delivery among rural Indian women. *Plos One*, 12(12), e0190117.

Goudar, S. S., Goco, N., Somannavar, M. S., Vernekar, S. S., Mallapur, A. A., Moore, J. L., ... & Goldenberg, R. L. (2015). Institutional deliveries and perinatal and neonatal mortality in Southern and Central India. *Reproductive Health*, *12*(2), 1–9.

International Conference on Population and Development (ICPD) in Cairo, Egypt, on 5–13 September 1994.

Jungari, S., & Paswan, B. (2019). What he knows about her and how it affects her? Husband's knowledge of pregnancy complications and maternal health care utilization among tribal population in Maharashtra, India. *BMC Pregnancy and Childbirth*, 19(1), 70.

Kumar, G. A., Dandona, R., Chaman, P., Singh, P., & Dandona, L. (2014). A population-based study of neonatal mortality and maternal care utilization in the Indian state of Bihar. *BMC Pregnancy and Childbirth*, *14*(1), 1–10.

Kifle, M. M., Kesete, H. F., Gaim, H. T., Angosom, G. S., & Araya, M. B. (2018). Health facility or home delivery? Factors influencing the choice of delivery place among mothers living in rural communities of Eritrea. *Journal of Health, Population and Nutrition*, *37*(1), 1–15.

Lehmann, U., Friedman, I., & Sanders, D. (2004). Review of the utilisation and effectiveness of community-based health workers in Africa. *Global Health Trust, Joint Learning Initiative on Human Resources for Health and Development (JLI), JLI Working Paper*, *4*, 1–44.

Leone, T., James, K. S., & Padmadas, S. S. (2013). The burden of maternal health care expenditure in India: multilevel analysis of national data. *Maternal and Child Health Journal*, *17*(9), 1622–1630.

Mishra, S., & Mohanty, S. K. (2019). Out-of-pocket expenditure and distress financing on institutional delivery in India. *International Journal for Equity in Health*, *18*(1), 1–15.

National Family Health Survey in India, NFHS-4, 2015–2016, IIPS Mumbai

National Population Policy (2000). Dept. of Family Welfare, Ministry of Health and Family Welfare, Government of India.

Navaneetham, Kannan & Dharmalingam, A. (2002). Utilization of Maternal Health Care Services in Southern India. *Social Science & Medicine Part D Medical Geography* 55. 1849–69. https://doi.org/10.1016/S0277-9536(01)00313-6.

Nesbitt, R. C., Lohela, T. J., Soremekun, S., Vesel, L., Manu, A., Okyere, E., ... & Gabrysch, S. (2016). The influence of distance and quality of care on place of delivery in rural Ghana. *Scientific Reports*, *6*(1), 1–8.

Rutaremwa, G., Wandera, S. O., Jhamba, T., Akiror, E., & Kiconco, A. (2015). Determinants of maternal health services utilization in Uganda. *BMC Health Services Research*, *15*(1), 1–8.

Singh, A., Kumar, A., & Pranjali, P. (2014a). Utilization of maternal healthcare among adolescent mothers in urban India: evidence from DLHS-3. *PeerJ*, *2*, e592.

Singh, A., Pallikadavath, S., Ram, F., & Alagarajan, M. (2014b). Do antenatal care interventions improve neonatal survival in India?. *Health Policy and Planning*, *29*(7), 842–848.

Skordis-Worrall, J., Pace, N., Bapat, U. *et al.* Maternal and neonatal health expenditure in Mumbai slums (India): A cross sectional study. *BMC Public Health* 11, 150 (2011). https://doi.org/10.1186/1471-2458-11-150

UNICEF. (2019). UNICEF Data: Monitoring the situation of children and women. Retrieved June 10, 2020, from data.unicef.org: https://data.unicef.org/topic/maternal-health/antenatal-care

World Health Organisation (2020): https://www.who.int/news-room/fact-sheets/detail/newborns-reducing-mortality

World Health Organisation (WHO). *Alma Ata Declaration.* Geneva: World Health Organization; 1978.

Zeng, L., Cheng, Y., Dang, S., Yan, H., Dibley, M. J., Chang, S., & Kong, L. (2008). Impact of micronutrient supplementation during pregnancy on birth weight, duration of gestation, and perinatal mortality in rural western China: double blind cluster randomised controlled trial. *BMJ*, *337*.

CHAPTER 5

Quality of Care at Public Health Institutions: Identifying Gaps

Introduction

Newborn survival has been one of the key global health agendas prioritised both in the MDGs and in the SDGs. For the past many years, there has been an overarching focus on increasing the number of facility births and skilled birth attendants to reduce maternal and newborn deaths. As a result of a number of concerted efforts, institutional delivery has gained momentum in the country and has increased manifold in Bihar. Almost four-fifths of all deliveries are institutional in the state, which number was less than half until a decade ago. Neonatal mortality, on the other hand, is accompanied by a slower pace of decline. This indicates institutional deliveries may not be much protective against neonatal mortality unless emphasis should be placed on the quality of care (QoC) received during childbirth. Increasing evidences show that in low-income settings, poor quality of care results in higher maternal and neonatal mortality (Randive et al. 2013; Akachi and Kruk 2017) and up to 1.49 million maternal and newborn deaths and stillbirths could be averted annually with improved QoC (Graham et al. 2016). Utilisation of higher quality of services not only lowers newborn mortality, but also improves subsequent school performance, which is critical to future labour productivity (Van der Gaag 2010).

Historically, health system of low-income countries focuses mostly on expansion in the physical infrastructure instead of improving the quality of

S. R. Mahapatro, *Towards Newborn Survival*,
https://doi.org/10.1007/978-981-19-3417-9_5

healthcare. Inaccessibility of health services, distance, socio-cultural differences, and economic constraints is only a part of the problem of utilisation of healthcare services. An ample amount of evidence shows that even after making it to a health facility, people face difficulties with receiving adequate and good quality services due to factors related to the health personnel, equipment, hygiene, and other factors like shortage of beds, unavailability of drugs, long waiting time, and so on. With the launching of NRHM, Indian public health system made efforts to improve the quality of healthcare resources which were long ignored earlier. It is evident from Chap. 3 that effective facility care at birth not only acts as an enabler of institutional delivery but is also paramount to reducing neonatal deaths in the state. This finding is in line with other studies that show that due to the failure on the part of facilities to provide quality care, facility delivery does not confer any survival benefits on mother and baby (Gabrysch et al. 2019). Hence, providing high-quality care around childbirth is crucial to reduce adverse birth outcomes (Akachi and Kruk 2017). Recent evidences indicate that poor quality of care at primary healthcare facilities—the first point of contact with the health system—not only jeopardises the health of mothers and newborns but also erodes trust, resulting in people bypassing health facilities and potentially putting the entire healthcare system and population at risk (Kruk et al. 2018a). Identification of gaps in the provision of services, thus, is significant to guide the policy makers to take appropriate actions to overcome the challenges involved in providing quality care.

The state of Bihar faces various challenges in the provision of quality healthcare given the weak public health system and resource crunch to improve it. Though the initiatives under NRHM spurred progress, there is still a deficiency in health infrastructure in the state. It is evident from Chap. 3 that the pace of improvement in health infrastructure, in terms of availability of facilities, trained medical staff, and other material resources, is lower than the increase in the demand for healthcare services. In conjunction with the supply-side challenges, the inhibitors embedded in the complex social system of the state—as reflected in the attitudes and behaviour of the staff—likely influence the delivery of services. The complex interplay of these forces operating together influences the quality of maternal and newborn services offered, especially in public institutions. Given the state of healthcare and the complex social system of Bihar, in this chapter, I seek to offer insights into the quality of services provided at facilities from the perspective of the users and identify the barriers to improved care.

Measuring the quality of care for mothers and newborns is multidimensional and conceptually complex. The World Health Organization (2016) defines quality of MNH care as 'the degree to which maternal and newborn health services (for individuals and population) increase the likelihood of timely, appropriate care for the purpose of achieving desired outcomes that are both consistent with current professional knowledge and take into account the preferences and aspirations of individual women and their families'. Quality-assessment studies usually measure one of three types of outcomes: Medical outcomes, costs, or client's satisfaction. While medical outcomes and costs are linked to the provision of care, client's satisfaction is associated with perceptions/satisfaction of the clients with the services. Though patients' perception of quality is an important measure, it is influenced by their individual characteristics (Zaslavsky et al. 2000). Hence, researchers also rely on evidence-based quality criteria such as the provision of services as per the normative standards. Due to the limits of health outcomes to measure the quality of services, often healthcare structure and process features are assessed as indirect indicators of quality (Williams 1994). Within the classic framework of structure-process-outcomes, the newborn survival and its linkages with quality of services are guided by these two aspects of quality framework: *Structure* as in the organisational and professional resources associated with the provision of healthcare, and *Process* as in how the care given is measured through the experience of care (Donabedian 1980).

Clients' Satisfaction with Quality of Care (Experiences of Care)

One of the measures of Quality of Care (QoC) is an assessment of the service recipients' satisfaction with and perception of the quality of health services (Fisher 1971; Barnett 1995). The experiences of women while accessing ANC as well as at the hospital during their stay for delivery provide glimpses into the effectiveness of facility care. Poor service quality offered at ANC period may influence the expected mode of delivery and impede further service utilisation. More than three-quarters of service users in the survey discontinued ANC, and the figure was significantly higher among those who availed the services from Anganwadi Centres.

Approximately one in five women were dissatisfied with the quality of service at AWCs, while the level of dissatisfaction was lower for facility care. Despite the provision of free care and the attempts to universalise ANC services, dissatisfaction with the services received pushed women to discontinue accessing ANC. This is a reflection of the poor quality of services at institutions. Evidences in this regard suggest that satisfaction of patients, although highly individualistic, depends, by and large, upon the supply-side factors related to the interpersonal skills of the service provider and the commodity elements in the setting where the services are provided (Aldana et al. 2001).

To assess the quality of services and its implication on neonatal health, patients were asked to describe their experience during their stay in a facility. Questions asked were related to the waiting period, staff behaviour and support, availability of staff, availability of skilled personnel, cleanliness, functional equipment, privacy, counselling on postnatal care, and so on. The responses for each of the indicators were classified as: Very good, good, bad, and very bad. Among the indicators, waiting time (18 per cent) and negative approach of healthcare providers (6.9 per cent) were identified as major difficulties to client satisfaction (Fig. 5.1). Long waiting period was cited by the highest number of women in West Champaran (25 per cent), followed by Madhubani (22.8 per cent) and Kishanganj (20.8 per cent). Following that, disrespectful treatment was cited by

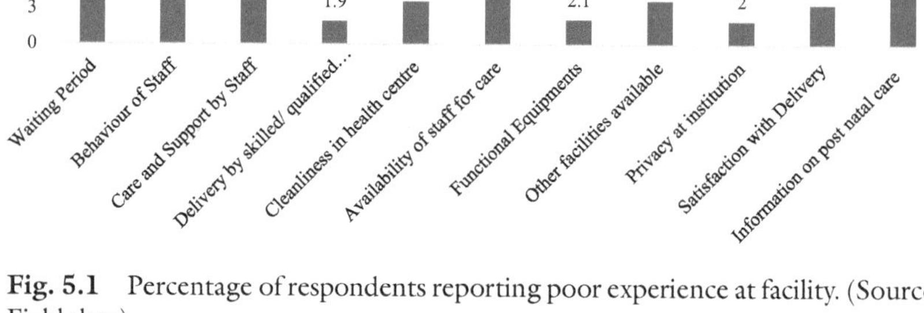

Fig. 5.1 Percentage of respondents reporting poor experience at facility. (Source: Field data)

members of staff from 3.6 per cent women in Kishanganj to 14 per cent in Muzaffarpur. Almost 5 per cent of the respondents were dissatisfied due to care deficiency and staff unavailability.

The attitude of service providers, which is also linked to long waiting times, was found to be a major barrier to facility delivery and newborn care. Lack of respectful care from service providers may lead to dissatisfaction with the health system, diminishing the likelihood of seeking antenatal care and delivery and postnatal services (WHO 2005). Prejudice of healthcare providers, experienced in the form of rude and disrespectful behaviour and ignorance towards the poor and the marginalised, acts as a barrier to the use of MNH services (Kruk et al. 2018b). In our study, the mode of delivery had changed to home delivery for a quarter of the respondents who had previously endured abuse or had perceived the behaviour of the service providers as abusive in the facility. Studies in African countries have found that abusive treatment resulted in adverse consequences for the reproductive life as reflected in an increased risk of birth complications, post-traumatic stress disorder, and the like (Rance et al. 2013).

The interaction between the supply- and demand-side factors weaves complicated relationships that influence the quality-of-service delivery around childbirth and during the stay. In the survey, it was observed that the client-provider relationship varied according to the socioeconomic status and that the marginalised were the most disadvantaged. For instance, long waiting time, as an indicator of dissatisfaction, was reported by 22 per cent of women from the poorest class, while only 10 per cent of women from the richest class expressed dissatisfaction due to waiting time. Likewise, dissatisfaction with services was higher among poor women (38 per cent) than rich women (28 per cent). While around 31 per cent women from the marginalised community reported poor quality of care in public facilities, the corresponding figure was 28 per cent for upper-caste women.

While explaining the behaviour of the staff towards her, one respondent from Rohtas district reported feeling like she had lost her dignity. She explained her experience as:

> *The midwife would not listen to me, and I was verbally abused. I was in pain and crying because of that. The midwife said to me: 'If you could enjoy sex, why can't you bear the pain?'* (In the local language: 'sone me sauk lagta he; ab bacha karne me dard lagta he').

She further reported that the staff kept the pregnant women on the floor for some time.

One of the respondents went to a facility but returned and delivered the baby at home. She narrated her experience as follows:

> *I went to the facility with the belief that I would get better care. I had to return because I did not get appropriate care, and no one would listen to me. I went on to give birth at home. Unless I have a serious problem, I will not visit health facility nor will I recommend it to anyone. I have a strong faith in the rural doctors (informal care providers); they treat us well. Three-four days after the delivery, the baby got any eye infection. The doctor did a check-up. I acted on his advice, and the baby was cured.* (Manju Devi, 35, Nalanda)

The woman, however, was not aware of breastfeeding and postnatal care practices and no frontline worker visited her.

Another case from Nalanda revealed:

> *The doctor was negligent at the time of the delivery; so it was the ANM who had to conduct the procedure. The ANM did not have complete knowledge regarding the health problems of the mother and the child due to which they both suffered. The baby was convulsive the day after birth and had difficulty breathing. Medicines had to be purchased from outside the hospital. The mother and the child were referred to a private hospital when the baby's condition did not improve, and the baby had to be put on the ventilator. They were sent to another hospital the next day, where the baby was kept admitted for 5 days and given appropriate treatment. Even post discharge, the baby was unwell for another 15–20 days.*

The stories related by women of their experience with childbirth at facilities provide glimpses of the quality of service, necessitating further attention to bring about improvements in its supply.

A composite index of QoC was constructed considering all the indicators that measured a patient's satisfaction with the services received. The score value of the index was divided into three groups: Poor, good, and better. QoC below the mean score was classified as poor quality. Good quality was where, irrespective of all indicators, the response was good, while in the case of better QoC, the responses were mainly good/very good. This assessment was based on the opinions of the respondents and was not verified by an actual visit to the specific health facilities where the woman delivered. The average score of the QoC was 63, representing that the quality of care was good; this was slightly higher in private facilities (66.3 per cent) than the public ones (62 per cent). On an average, around four in every ten women experienced poor quality of care during their stay in public facilities. Women in West Champaran (37 per cent) experienced poor QoC while quality of services was reported better mostly in Jehanabad (74 per cent). The quality of services offered at private facilities was reported as relatively better but had not varied much from public facility.

Provision of Care Around Childbirth and Hospital Stay

The perception of care received around childbirth and during the stay in the postnatal period is a reflection of the adherence to the standard procedures of healthcare, or it may be individually driven. In the survey, a standard set of questions was incorporated to assess the quality of service, which served to reflect the features and functioning of the health system. The questions pertained to duration of stay, waiting time, tests conducted, postnatal advice, ambulance facility, availability of free drugs and medicines, and the like (Table 5.1).

Women who delivered at a facility were usually accompanied by community workers or other family members. At the facility, they had to wait, on an average, 20 minutes merely to receive the registration slip. Around 30 per cent of respondents recalled they had to wait more than 20 minutes to be attended to by a health personnel and to receive the registration slip. As stated above, experiencing long waiting times is a major constraint to receive timely and appropriate care. The length of stay, again, is a widely used indicator of quality-of-service delivery and the health outcomes. According to the WHO guidelines, the minimum duration of stay after delivery in a health facility should be 24 hours to 48 hours so that the mother and the child can get timely interventions and recover well if any complication arises. In the survey, a majority of the women—almost three-fourths—who had delivered in a public facility stayed less than 24 hours, whereas the scenario was the reverse in the case of private facilities. The exit interview of women who delivered in public facilities also showed that the mean duration of stay in the hospital after delivery was only 11 hours.

A respondent who had a facility delivery shared her experience thus:

After delivering the baby, I stayed at the hospital only for four hours. After measuring the weight of the baby and giving her an injection, the medical staff

Table 5.1 Service delivery during hospital stay

Details of hospital stay	*Public*	*Private*
Duration of stay in the hospital		
More than 24 hours	27.3	71.4
C-section	76.8	95.6
Average duration of stay (hrs)	10.6	–
Time taken for registration (in minutes)	20	18
Reasons for leaving the hospital within 24 hrs		
Doctor/ANM suggested	93.8	95.4
No proper infrastructure	1.5	0.4
No family support/suggestions	2.4	1.2
Neglect/improper behaviour of staff	0.5	1.3
No food/drugs	1.9	2.5
Other	1.9	1.7
Tests done before leaving hospital (N = 1881)		
BP measurement	39.8	64.9
Pulse rate measurement	34.9	60.8
Body temperature	10.2	27.8
Urine test	1.7	8.8
Other	0.1	0.7
No	57.8	31.2
Advise about care & nutrition	48	83.8
Re-examination of baby before discharge	38.8	77.8
Recommended for PNC visit	31.7	64.4
Paid user charges	21.1	78.5
Ambulance facility	25.9	3
Free Drop up facility	37.6	4.2
Free medicine	66.6	3.1
Free blood test	19.6	1.6

Source: Field data

> *asked me to leave the hospital as there was a shortage of beds.* (Priyanka Devi, Muzaffarpur District)

A disproportionate share of women who had undergone a C-section stayed for more than 24 hours, both in public and private facilities. Several factors are reportedly associated with length of stay, including readiness of the mother for discharge (clinical and perceived) (Nilsson et al. 2017).

Quality components were also important in determining the duration of stay in a public facility. The shortfall in the health infrastructure, due to high demand, and the high indirect expenditure pose challenges to longer hospital stays. Most of the women reported leaving the hospital at the suggestion of the doctor/ANM which is mainly intertwined with shortage of beds and staffs at facility. Due to the higher demand for beds than the hospital can meet, the patients are asked to leave just a few hours after birth. In public facilities, 2.4 per cent of women left the hospital due to lack of family support, while in private facilities, 2.5 per cent of women left due to lack of food/drugs. In terms of shortfall in sub-centres and CHCs, Bihar ranks the highest among all states (RHS 2019). The state is in need of almost 43 per cent additional PHCs. Although more than half of the PHCs function 24*7, which is comparatively higher than many states, more than half of them are out of OTs, labour rooms, and beds.

The Janani Shishu Suraksha Karyakram (JSSK), launched in 2011, provides service guarantees in the form of entitlement to pregnant women and sick newborns and infants. This includes free to and fro transportation between home and institution, diet, diagnostics, drugs, other consumables, and also blood transfusion if required. Despite this, almost one in five respondents paid user charges for admission/other services in public facilities. Around three-quarters of respondents in public hospitals received free drugs, and one-fifth had a free blood test. In the rural areas of Bihar, as observed in earlier chapters, distance to the facility, inadequate transportation, and higher cost featured as important reasons affecting the decision to seek medical help. An easy access to government transportation and referral services increases institutional deliveries (Prinja et al. 2013). In the study area, only a quarter of respondents had access to ambulance services and 38 per cent received free drop facility home. Poor transportation facilities greatly affect timely access to healthcare services and, consequently, mother and child health outcomes. In private hospitals, most of the service deliveries are guided by the individual motive, and people make their own arrangements for taking care of the mother and the newborn.

In keeping with the guidelines of the Universal Immunization Programme and now the Intensified Mission Indradhanush, of the many scheduled vaccines, BCG and zero OPV are administered soon after birth. In this study, almost 64 per cent of the respondents reported having the knowledge that a newborn requires vaccination at birth and the coverage was almost universal. Recommendations by doctors/nurses regarding postnatal practices or health check-ups before discharge are a kind of behavioural change intervention and also an indicator to assess the quality-of-service delivery. Less than half of the women who had delivered in a public facility reported receiving advice on the health and nutrition of the baby or having been re-examined or having received postnatal check-ups (48 per cent, 40 per cent, and 32 per cent respectively). The facts presented above show that the health facilities do not follow 100 per cent compliance with the JSSK guidelines.

Discussion

The commendable increase in institutional delivery as the data reveals has not translated into a desired reduction in newborn mortality in Bihar. The study finds moving from a staggering focus of increasing facility birth to effective facility delivery with good quality services is inevitable for newborn survival. This chapter of the book provides an assessment of the gaps in quality of facility care through a recollection of the experiences of the patients and an evaluation of the services offered against the standard norms. The issues and challenges in the quality of care were mainly assessed through the supply-side determinants, inherent to the health system. The findings show that the state is a long way off from achieving the standards of good quality of care. The ground realities had the impression that due to lack of supply of services and unwelcoming staff attitude and discriminatory treatment, health facilities often struggle in satisfying the users' need. Long waiting time, as an important reason for patients' dissatisfaction, is associated with the availability of staff and equipment and the management of the premises in accordance with the needs of the facility. A healthy attitude of the providers towards the users helps build a relationship of trust in the health system.

The standard norms laid down by the Indian public health system are not followed in the health facilities. Length of stay was almost four times lower than the desired norm. While this may have been impacted by the personal attributes of the respondents, the supply of quality services in this context is also determinantal. Poor and inadequate supply of services is reflected in the poor provision of ambulance services and infrastructural deficiencies that facilitate institutional delivery. For instance, as presented in Chap. 3, only one-fifth of PHCs and CHCs of the state followed IPHS norms. It may be said that while an improvement in the health system has occurred with the implementation of NRHM, there is still plenty of scope to improve the quality of care.

For enhancing the use of health services and reducing adverse MNH outcomes, such health system crises require urgent solutions. Emphasis should be given on improving the compliance with the IPHS standards, monitoring the services regularly, and taking corrective actions to overcome the structural bottlenecks that impede the provision of a better quality of health services. Greater transparency and innovative approaches may fill the gaps in providing quality service. Improvements in service delivery will alter the perception of the patients towards the quality of care at the facilities and act as a driving force for an increased use of MNH health services. For addressing the barriers for effective facility care, the findings call for identifying the possible levels of intervention as well as evolving strategies for interventions.

References

Akachi, Y., & Kruk, M. E. (2017). Quality of care: measuring a neglected driver of improved health. *Bulletin of the World Health Organization*, *95*(6), 465.

Aldana, J. M., Piechulek, H., & Al-Sabir, A. (2001). Client satisfaction and quality of health care in rural Bangladesh. *Bulletin of the World Health Organization*, *79*, 512–517.

Barnett, B. (1995). Women's views influence use. *Network (Research Triangle Park, NC)*, *16*(1), 14–18.

Donabedian, A. (1980). Basic approaches to assessment: structure, process and outcome. *The Definition of Quality and Approaches to Its Assessment: Explorations in Quality Assessment and Monitoring*, *1*, 77–128.

Fisher, A. W. (1971). Patients' evaluation of outpatient medical care. *Academic Medicine*, *46*(3), 238–44.

Gabrysch, S., Nesbitt, R. C., Schoeps, A., Hurt, L., Soremekun, S., Edmond, K., ... Campbell, O. M. (2019). Does facility birth reduce maternal and perinatal mortality in Brong Ahafo, Ghana? A secondary analysis using data on 119 244 pregnancies from two cluster-randomised controlled trials. *The Lancet Global Health*, *7*(8), e1074–e1087.

Graham, W., Woodd, S., Byass, P., Filippi, V., Gon, G., Virgo, S., ... & Singh, S. (2016). Diversity and divergence: the dynamic burden of poor maternal health. *The Lancet*, *388*(10056), 2164–2175.

Kruk, M. E., Gage, A. D., Arsenault, C., Jordan, K., Leslie, H. H., Roder-DeWan, S., ... Pate, M. (2018a). High-quality health systems in the Sustainable Development Goals era: time for a revolution. *The Lancet Global Health*, *6*(11), e1196–e1252.

Kruk, M. E., Kujawski, S., Mbaruku, G., Ramsey, K., Moyo, W., & Freedman, L. P. (2018b). Disrespectful and abusive treatment during facility delivery in Tanzania: a facility and community survey. *Health Policy and Planning*, *33*(1), e26–e33.

Nilsson, I. M., Kronborg, H., Knight, C. H., & Strandberg-Larsen, K. (2017). Early discharge following birth—What characterises mothers and newborns?. *Sexual & Reproductive Healthcare*, *11*, 60–68.

Prinja, S., Manchanda, N., Mohan, P. et al. (2013). Cost of neonatal intensive care delivered through district level public hospitals in India. *Indian Pediatr* 50, 839–846. https://doi.org/10.1007/s13312-013-0234-6

Rance, S., McCourt, C., Rayment, J., Mackintosh, N., Carter, W., Watson, K., & Sandall, J. (2013). Women's safety alerts in maternity care: is speaking up enough?. *BMJ Quality & Safety*, *22*(4), 348–355.

Randive, B., Diwan, V., & De Costa, A. (2013). India's conditional cash transfer programme (the JSY) to promote institutional birth: is there an association between institutional birth proportion and maternal mortality?. *PloS One*, *8*(6), e67452.

Rural Health Statistics Report 2019–20, National Rural Health Mission, Ministry of Health and Family Welfare, Government of India.

Van der Gaag, J. (2010). From child development to human development. In *Development and Prevention of Behaviour Problems* (pp. 231–242). Psychology Press.

Williams, B. (1994). Patient satisfaction: a valid concept?. *Social Science & Medicine*, *38*(4), 509–516.

World Health Organization. (2016). *Standards for improving quality of maternal and newborn care in health facilities.*

World Health Organization. (2005). *The World health report: 2005: make every mother and child count.* World Health Organization.

Zaslavsky, A. M., Hochheimer, J. N., Schneider, E. C., Cleary, P. D., Seidman, J. J., McGlynn, E. A., ... Epstein, A. M. (2000). Impact of sociodemographic case mix on the HEDIS measures of health plan quality. *Medical Care*, 981–992.

CHAPTER 6

Newborn Care Practices and Barriers to Service Utilisation

Introduction

In recent times, Bihar has seen a dramatic decline in infant and child mortality, whereas the fall in NMR has been relatively slower and stagnant for years. Almost three-quarters of infant deaths occur in the neonatal period in many states of India; however, the share is disproportionately high in Odisha and Bihar (79.7 per cent and 78.7 per cent). In this study, the known causes of neonatal deaths made up 70 per cent of the total deaths. While over half of these deaths were due to prematurity/low birth weight and birth asphyxia—which generally require skilled intrapartum care—almost a third of the deaths were attributed to infection/diarrhoea/diseases. Such deaths occurred after discharge from the hospital and could have been prevented by appropriate postnatal care. Postnatal care deals with issues pertaining to the mother and the baby from birth up to six weeks (WHO 2014). Over two-thirds of newborn deaths in the study area occurred during the first week of birth. An increase in the medicalisation of childbirth alone, therefore, is not sufficient since it is the neonatal period which is the riskiest for the newborns.

The highest risk of newborn death occurs around the time of childbirth and within the first few weeks after birth; hence, the immediate postpartum period is thus extremely critical (Singh et al. 2012). PNC is an important link in the continuum of care for both mother and child and is cost-effective in reducing neonatal mortality in low-income settings

S. R. Mahapatro, *Towards Newborn Survival*,
https://doi.org/10.1007/978-981-19-3417-9_6

(Kumar et al. 2008). PNC interventions prevent newborn complications that arise during delivery, such as sepsis, meningitis, pneumonia, and diarrhoea, and include follow-up care for all newborns, especially those who are born premature (WHO 2014). The postnatal period is a critical transition time for a woman and her newborn physiologically, emotionally, and socially (MacArthur et al. 2002) and a time of behavioural transition, representing an opportunity to promote healthy behaviours that have benefits beyond the neonatal period (Lawn and Kerber 2006).

Realising the significance of postnatal care, the Home-Based Newborn Care programme was launched in India in 2011 following the strategy implemented by Bang and others in their study in Maharashtra. The significance of PNC has been reiterated in the 'Every Newborn Action Plan (2014)' and the 'India Newborn Action Plan', with emphasis on the critical periods of labour, birth, and the first week of life as time points when interventions can make the maximum impact on saving newborn lives. Evidence shows that multiple home visits by trained community-level health workers in Maharashtra and Uttar Pradesh reduced neonatal death by 62 per cent and 54 per cent respectively (Bang et al. 1999; Kumar et al. 2008). Such cost-effective community-based interventions are aimed at improving maternal knowledge of postnatal services and at bringing about change in the traditional practices associated with postnatal care. Home visits of the community workers to advise on the health and hygiene of newborns and mothers, together with an appropriate follow-up, promote preventive and curative care and help reduce neonatal mortality.

Despite the consensus that PNC interventions should be intensified for newborn survival, their coverage and utilisation are low in India, specifically in Bihar. Although the increase in facility delivery should have made it easy for the frontline workers to do follow-up visits, the fact is that it does not induce utilisation of postnatal services in the state. Only 27 per cent of women visited a facility for the health assessment of the baby within two days of birth (NFHS 2015–2016). Evidences from low-income countries like Uganda and Zambia, on the concomitant factors of postnatal services, have shown the suboptimal coverage of postnatal care services attributable to both demand- and supply-side factors such as age, education, poverty, cultural beliefs, location, quality of care, and communication with and training of healthcare workers (Kyomuhendo 2003; Raven et al. 2007; Singh et al. 2012).

Postnatal interventions proved to be effective in newborn survival presented in Chap. 3. While there is a growing recognition that the prevalence of harmful practices underlies the deaths of newborns, PNC provides an opportunity to correct the myths and misconceptions; bring about a behavioural change in newborn care practices. Given this, the present chapter attempts to explore the coverage and quality of postnatal care and explores the barriers to essential newborn care practices in the state.

Utilisation of Postnatal Services by Place of Delivery

The lower utilisation of postnatal services continues to be a major concern for the public health system of Bihar. The deep-rooted cultural norms along with fragile health services impede the use of PNC. A significant proportion of mothers in the study returned home within 24 hours of childbirth, three out of five mothers were discharged within 24 hours, primarily on the recommendation of the physicians/ANMs and could not carry out postnatal follow-up. About 10 per cent of respondents who had delivered at a facility recalled that their babies had not undergone postnatal examination at all. Postnatal counselling at the time of discharge is hardly done in public facilities. Only three in ten women were advised to visit a facility during the postnatal period. This was evident from the number of postnatal visits, with limited to fewer than one-fifth of the respondents, the number of visits being higher in the case of deliveries at private facilities (32 per cent) than those in public facilities (17 per cent) and home deliveries (13.4 per cent).

The suboptimum use of PNC in the study area highlights the importance of home-based newborn practices delivered by community workers. The increasing importance of HBNC is especially relevant in states like Bihar where a substantial portion of deliveries (more than one-fifth) occurs outside formal health facilities. These births required adequate care because only about a trained birth attendant delivered 5 per cent of home births. Home deliveries were particularly higher in underserved areas, resource-crunch families, and among the marginalised. Although continuous efforts have been made for the universalisation of postnatal care, the coverage is likely influenced by the socioeconomic context of the family as discussed in the next section.

The socioeconomic differentials in PNC as observed in the field reveals, education of woman and her husband, improved economic status, and knowledge of and exposure to outside world were the factors facilitating the use of postnatal care. Urban mothers went to a health facility slightly more frequently than rural mothers, while the number of visits by community workers was higher in rural areas.

Status of Newborn Care Practices

The association of postnatal indicators and neonatal mortality, presented in Chap. 3, underscores the importance of PNC in newborn survival. The World Health Organization recommends that postnatal care for newborns should include exclusive breastfeeding, warming of the infant, hygienic care of the umbilical cord, and timely identification of danger signs such as bleeding and infection with referral and treatment (WHO 1998).

Postnatal care practices are the easiest, most economical and vital response to newborn health and protect from many childhood illnesses. The service delivery modes for postnatal care include family, community, outreach services, and facility-based care. This section explains the status of immediate and essential postnatal care practices, which, if followed, increase the chances of survival. Such interventions can address the main causes of neonatal mortality. Table 6.1 presents the coverage of newborn care indicators by place of delivery.

Table 6.1 Immediate care given to the newborns according to the place of delivery

Type of care given	*Public*	*Private*	*Home*	*Total*
Immediate care				
Skin-to-skin care	87.5	76.4	60.0	79.1
Skin-to-skin care (within a minute)	43.4	34.4	24.5	34.4
Not wrapped without being wiped	38.1	36	40.4	38.2
Bath after 24 hours of birth	77.5	76.4	73.0	76.3
Applied anything on the umbilical cord	64.0	62.1	62.7	63.3
No hygiene at place of birth	3.5	1.2	12.9	5.2
Early initiation of breastfeeding	84	38	79	74
Colostrum feeding	91.6	78.4	86.1	87.7
Prelacteal feeding	4.0	14.3	11	8
Daily care				
Skin-to-skin care	51	53	48	50
Baby bath	61.5	56	58	60
Cord care	53	54	49	52
Eye care	31	34	29	31
Hand wash/hygiene	38	40	29	36
N	1358	523	503	2384

Source: Field data

Skin-to-Skin Care

Early skin-to-skin care (an important part of kangaroo mother care) is a process that involves placing a bare newborn on the bare breast of the mother (without any barrier, i.e. without the mother's gown or a towel) and covering the infant with a blanket to keep it dry and warm. The process should be started immediately after birth or shortly after birth, with the baby remaining on the mother's chest until at least the end of the first breastfeeding session (Moore et al. 2016). Giving skin-to-skin care is like a natural incubator for the child as it provides warmth similar to what it receives in the mother's womb. It benefits both the baby and the mother eventually by building a healthier bond between them, reducing maternal/newborn anxiety, enhancing child cognitive development, and facilitating mother-child reciprocity (Moore et al. 2016). Around four among five newborns, in this study, were given skin-to-skin care, and 34.4 per cent were given early skin-to-skin care within one minute after birth.

Thermal Care

Bathing of the baby should be delayed, with priority given to skin-to-skin care, both in case of normal and caesarean deliveries. Delay in baby bath gives the newborn the time to acclimatise to the new environment and reduces the chances of pneumonia. It even reduces the risk of infection, stabilises infant blood sugar, improves maternal-infant bonding, and improves breastfeeding. Bathing causes crying, stress, and the release of stress hormones. That leads to a drop in the blood sugar levels. However, taking care of hygiene is essential to prevent both mother and newborn from various infections.

Thermal care showed an encouraging prevalence, with almost three-quarters of respondents reporting having delayed baby birth until after 24 hours. Regarding the birthplace hygiene, lack of hygiene was found more commonly in the case of home delivery (13 per cent) than facility delivery. Approximately 40 per cent babies were immediately wrapped, without being wiped off, before the delivery of the placenta (Table 6.1).

Cord Care

Care of the cord is necessary to keep the baby away from infections as the cord is a common portal of entry for invasive pathogenic bacteria (Mullany et al. 2008). Suggestions on cord care by ASHAs/ANMs were reported by only 34.2 per cent women in the study. More than two-thirds of respondents applied gentian violet on the cord stump for faster healing, purchased mainly from local shops. Information on the quality of the violet and the manner in which it should be applied should be incorporated into the awareness campaigns.

Early Initiation of Breastfeeding

Breastfeeding reduces neonatal death and safeguards infant development. Around one-fifth of the neonatal deaths can be prevented if there is an early initiation of breastfeeding and exclusive breastfeeding (Jones et al. 2003) as doing so reduces neonatal infections (sepsis, pneumonia, tetanus, and diarrhoea) (Mullany et al. 2008). According to a study, babies are more alert during the first 60 minutes of birth, and if put to mother's breast within this period, the chances of early initiation of breastfeeding increase, giving the babies neuron-developmental advantages (Georgieff et al. 1997). Recognising the significance of breast milk on newborn health, the Government of India started a programme in 2016 to promote exclusive breastfeeding. In the study, initiation of breastfeeding within the first hour of birth was reported by 74 per cent women. The prevalence of early breastfeeding initiation was 84 per cent in the case of delivery in a public facility and 79 per cent in the case of home delivery. Around two-fifths of deliveries in a private facility (38 per cent) were associated with an early initiation, which was lower perhaps due to the greater number of C-section deliveries.

Colostrum and Prelacteal feeding

Colostrum is a vital component of the breast milk. It is important for the immune system (Godhia and Patel 2013) and is a life-saving nutrient. In traditional settings, however, the myths that prevail keep the newborn devoid of the colostrum even though it serves as the first immunisation (Chellaiyan et al. 2020). In the Indian society, it is customary to give a newborn prelacteal feed before initiating breastfeeding (Pathi 2005; Chaturvedi et al. 2007). This practice is a barrier to exclusive breastfeeding and increases the risk of infection, deaths, diarrhoea, and acute respiratory illnesses (UNICEF 2016). Although various healthcare interventions have attempted to address this issue, overcoming it has, nevertheless, proven to be a challenge for the state. The practice was observed in the case of approximately one-tenth of respondents (8 per cent) and was higher in the case of home delivery (11 per cent) compared to institutional delivery (7 per cent). The prevalence of prelacteal feeding was higher and that of feeding colostrum lower in private facilities because most of the women had undergone C-section deliveries. The most used prelacteal feed in the state was cow milk/powder milk (72.2 per cent), followed by honey and water (9.3 per cent). Honey and water is a commonly used prelacteal food in the rural areas of other states such as West Bengal (Mandal et al. 2007). A majority of the newborns received prelacteal food and were not given colostrum due to an illness (43 per cent), or the breast milk was delayed due to cultural practices (37 per cent).

Daily care routines were practiced by more than half of the respondents, though eye care and hand wash/hygiene were practiced by much fewer respondents in the study area. Irrespective of all the indicators, use of postnatal care was less prevalent in the case of home delivery than facility delivery.

Barriers to Postnatal Care Services

The Indian government has made efforts to implement home-based newborn care programmes for the universalisation of postnatal care practices. Such community-based interventions are deemed effective in improving the postnatal coverage. However, around one-third of respondents did not practise postnatal care as per standard norms. Low perceived value of postnatal visits (89.4 per cent) and lack of awareness (38 per cent) were found to be the major reasons for not visiting a facility. The low coverage of PNC reflects a gap in the continuum of MNH services. Several factors are associated with the non-utilisation of PNC. The social and institutional determinants of access to PNC vary depending on the socioeconomic and cultural environment. The following section addresses the range of reasons given by participants for the non-use of postnatal services.

Poor Perceived Need

In most parts of the state, specifically in the rural areas, the perception is that unless the newborn faces a serious medical problem and requires the intervention of doctors, it is not necessary to visit a hospital. Nine out of ten respondents, who did not practice postnatal care, believed that in the absence of a health problem, a newborn did not require any medical attention. In the study sites, over one-fifth of deliveries took place at home, and the women faced challenges in accessing PNC both from the community and from the institutions. The low perceived value of postnatal visits among the women resulted in the lower utilisation of the postnatal services.

Most of the respondents who had foregone facility visits for a check-up made similar observations as follows:

> *Unless a health problem arises, we do not go to a facility for the baby's check-up. I have a strong faith in the rural doctors (informal care providers). Three-four days after the delivery, my baby caught an eye infection. The rural doctor did a check-up. I followed his recommendations, and the baby was cured.*(Manju, Age 30, Nalanda)

The woman was unaware of breastfeeding and postnatal care practices, and no frontline worker had visited her.

Community Literacy/Lack of Awareness

Insufficient knowledge of PNC practices and their importance to newborn survival was found to obstruct the utilisation of postnatal care services. In the study, almost 38 per cent women reported lack of awareness as the reason for not practising PNC. Although the significance of colostrum feeding widespread, around 12 per cent of mothers had not fed colostrum to their newborn babies, of whom 5.4 per cent were unaware of its importance. Most of the women in the study area had no knowledge about the timing of breastfeeding. This implies that advice on breastfeeding during the prenatal visits had not been earnestly given. These findings are consistent with the findings of other studies in India and other low-income countries that lack of knowledge and awareness is the main reason why colostrum is discarded (Probandari et al. 2017; Randhawa et al. 2019).

The lack of awareness of the immediate postnatal care services was more concentrated in the lower economic class but, surprisingly, lower-caste women were more aware than their upper-caste counterparts. While 21 per cent of those from the poorest class did not practise skin-to-skin care immediately, the figure reduced to 11 per cent among the richest. Likewise, while the awareness of the importance of immediate skin-to-skin care was low among scheduled caste/tribe (14 per cent), it was lower still (16 per cent) among upper-caste women. Perhaps the inclusion of the Mahadalits in the healthcare programmes is beginning to pay dividends in the state.

Socioeconomic Inequality in Postnatal Care Practices

A clear class gradient was found with regard to the use of postnatal services much more than caste differences. Economic constraints, intersecting with knowledge gap, limit the use of postnatal care. On an average, the households had spent Rs. 973 to access and utilise postnatal care services. A huge economic inequality in PNC spending could be seen in the study area. The PNC expenditure of the poorest class as the study reveals is almost four times higher (33 per cent household budget) than the richest (8 per cent). The class differences in PNC spending indicate that the high burden of expenditure possibly discourages the poor from visiting facilities. While caste was not an impediment to accessing knowledge about immediate postnatal services, the caste differences were evident in the daily care practices. Perhaps the community-based interventions to raise awareness regarding PNC services are successful. The low use of postnatal services in the study area was, however, limited by behavioural constraints and other cultural practices.

Beliefs and Practices

The traditional practices, which vary from culture to culture in the country, possibly have a significant influence on newborn health. Traditional beliefs and cultural practices related to postnatal services have an impact on service utilisation such that they prevent improvements in neonatal health. In the study area, such practices prevented almost 8 per cent of women from breastfeeding within the first hour of birth. Some of the cultural practices—such as putting kajal in a baby's eyes and not bringing the baby into sunlight, assuming its harmful effect—influence the baby's growth and lead to infection. Many people believe that putting kajal in the eyes protects the baby against evil forces, unaware that it can have a harmful effect. In the study area, hygiene practices were recommended as a component of essential newborn care practices, but following those practices was uncommon. Over three-fifths (62 per cent) of women did not adopt such practices as their communities did not follow them.

Prelacteal feeding was practiced, and colostrum feeding was considered a harmful practice for the health of the baby. A majority of the respondents who spoke about giving yellow milk—the first milk—to the baby specified that they did so due to the promotion of evidence-based practices. Almost 12 per cent respondents, however, discarded the colostrum, and another 14 per cent (1.4 per cent of total respondents) discarded it on the belief of it not being good for newborn health. About 15 per cent of the women who did prelacteal feeding had the conception that colostrum was not good for the baby, which is why they initiated prelacteal food. They mainly fed honey, water, and cow milk. A study on a tribal community in Uttarakhand showed that undesirable cultural practices, such as late initiation of breastfeeding and avoidance of colostrum feeding, were still prevalent (Mukherjee and Venugopal 2018), mainly due to misconceptions (Randhawa et al. 2019). In the present study, most of the families reportedly applied a blue-coloured medicine, available in the local stores, for umbilical cord care, which showed that it was adopted as a community practice. Likewise, bathing was delayed for more than 24 hours, primarily due to the norm of celebrating the first ritual bath on the sixth day of birth (chatti). A few of the women reported that they cleaned their babies without properly bathing them until the sixth day as it is an auspicious day. Even in places where health services are offered, messengers of traditional cultural practices—like the elderly, the dais, and the village priests—pose challenges to the adoption of newborn care practices as per biomedical recommendations.

Shorter Length of Stay at Facilities

Longer length of stay in facilities is recognised as an opportunity for mothers of newborn babies to receive postnatal care education and prevent neonatal deaths caused due to immediate birth complications. The WHO recommends that newborns and mothers should remain in the facility for at least 24 to 48 hours after birth to reduce the risk of mortality and morbidity. With an increase in the length of the stay, the chances of survival of the newborn babies increase as they are monitored by a trained staff and receive appropriate care during the critical period. More than two-thirds (63 per cent) of neonates in the study area, who were discharged before 24 hours of birth, died compared with 37 per cent of those who stayed for more than 24 hours in the institutions. However, a significant discrepancy was observed in the actual and the recommended length of stay. Only 38 per cent of women stayed in a hospital for 24 hours or more after child birth. The determinants of the length of stay, as evident from various studies, are related to providers' characteristics, facilities available, need for stay, and characteristics of respondents and their children. In the study, lack of beds in the labour rooms and maternity wards forced the health officials to suggest that the clients leave the facility just after a few hours of child birth.

In this connection, one of the respondents had this to say:

> *I stayed there for four hours. After measuring the weight of the baby and giving him an injection, the medical staff told me to leave the hospital. The main reason was bed shortage.* (Priyanka Devi, Muzaffarpur)

Inadequate Pre-discharge Counselling

Postnatal education on neonatal care practices at the time of discharge from the hospital improves newborn care practices through behavioural changes as documented in various studies. Postnatal counselling on early identification of danger signs, breastfeeding, and care practices influences newborn health. The survey data showed a clear gap in the receipt of postnatal advices from facilities at the time of discharge. Only 32 per cent women who had delivered in a public facility were counselled about the postnatal services before leaving the hospital. Among the mothers who had been advised routine postnatal check-ups, over one-third (36.4 per cent) were not aware of all the components of postnatal services. These evidences clearly indicate that the counselling provided to women at the time of discharge was not adequate and did not properly communicate the importance of postnatal services. This compounded the lower use of postnatal services for mother and newborn.

Inadequate Reach of Interventions

To address the gaps in postnatal care services at facilities, the Ministry of Health and Family Welfare, Government of India, has implemented home-based newborn care programmes across the states of India, including Bihar. The aim is to strengthen the community linkages to continue the momentum towards a greater use of evidence-based newborn care practices. HBNC interventions serve to enhance the postnatal education of the family because although mother is the main caregiver, elderly members as messengers of traditional norms many times influence the postnatal care practices. The main provider under HBNC is the village health worker. ASHA, as a promoter of good health practices, has a prime role to play in creating awareness, providing counselling, and mobilising the community for service utilisation (Home Based Newborn Care, Operational Guidelines 2011). As per HBNC guidelines, home visits by health workers are as often as six times in the case of facility delivery and seven times in the case of home delivery within 42 days of the delivery.

The survey data suggests that such community-based interventions are effective in improving postnatal practices. In the study sites, visits by ASHA workers acted as a facilitating factor for promoting essential newborn care practices (Fig. 6.1). The figure depicts that skin-to-skin care, regular breastfeeding, care of umbilical cord, and hygiene practices were more common among those who were visited by ASHA workers. For

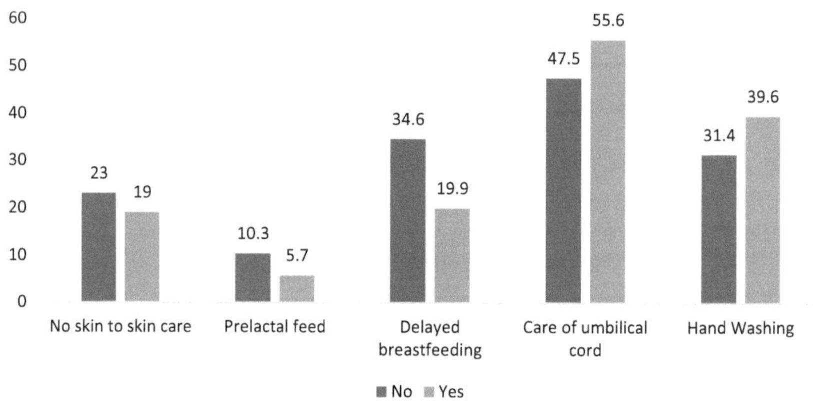

Fig. 6.1 Newborn care practices by ASHA worker visits. (Source: Field data)

instance, care of cord was practiced by 56 per cent of women who were visited by ASHA workers compared to 47.5 per cent of those who were not.

The role of ASHA workers in visiting and counselling the caregivers, however, was far from satisfactory in the study. While more than two-thirds of respondents stated that an ASHA worker had visited and advised them on postnatal practices, the visit of the health worker did not comply with the guidelines. The study revealed that ASHA workers visited a household a mere 1.3 times during the postnatal period. Of the total respondents, only 2.5 per cent had been visited five times or more, and the number was higher where there had been a delivery in a public facility (2.9 times) than in the case of home delivery (1.8 times). In this connection, studies show that although the role of ASHA workers in enhancing institutional delivery in the state cannot be undermined, gaps have been observed between institutional delivery and postpartum care. The data presented in the table reveals that the practice of ASHA workers giving suggestions on various components of PNC was relatively weak and that it was lower in the case of home delivery compared to facility delivery in public institutions. The prevalence of ASHA workers giving advice on skin-to-skin care, baby bathing, and so on was much lower than the other postnatal indicators (Table 6.2).

When asked about her reason for not availing services, one respondent stated:

> *I was never called for any meeting; hence I did not participate in any dissemination sessions. Due to lack of information, I never went to any public or private health institution.*

Table 6.2 Advice given by community workers regarding home-based PNC by place of delivery (in per cent)

Suggestions given by community workers	*Public*	*Private*	*Home*	*Total*	*N*
Breastfeeding	46.3	26.7	35.1	39.9	958
Skin-to-skin care	24.7	15.3	16.7	21.1	527
Baby bath	26.4	13.4	20.1	22.4	544
Keeping baby warm	21.6	11.4	14.8	18.1	446
Care of umbilical cord	40.5	22.0	28.7	34.2	817
Vaccination	54.3	36.6	47.3	49.2	1179

Source: Field data

The Government of India started the MAA or the 'Mothers Absolute Affection' programme in 2016 to enhance optimal breastfeeding practices, which include initiation of breastfeeding within one hour of birth and exclusive breastfeeding through counselling by ASHAs and ANMs. Nearly four-fifths of women who received breastfeeding counselling during the antenatal period breastfed their newborns and gave them colostrum in the first hour of birth. An increase in the frequency of ANM/ ASHA visits increased the newborns' propensity to be breastfed and to survive. A direct linear relationship was found between breastfeeding and the number of visits per ASHA worker over a 28-day period. Where ASHA visits were one or two in number, breastfeeding was done by 68 per cent of women. When the visits increased, the percentage of women who breastfed increased to over 80 per cent. In the survey, close to 6 per cent of respondents could not follow the suggestions made by the ASHA workers. The primary reason (62 per cent women) behind this was that the ASHA workers did not communicate to them about the newborn care practices well enough. However, based on their previous experience with child birth, there were women who availed facilities even without having received any ASHA worker's advice.

> *I was never told by any health worker to visit a facility for antenatal care or for a facility delivery. I am from a poor family; hence, I chose to visit a public facility. No ASHA worker ever visited me to provide suggestions regarding care practices. Since I already had the experience of child birth, I had the knowledge of care practices.* (Runu Kumari, scheduled caste, Nalanda)

However, she also followed the traditional care practice of putting kajal in the eyes of the newborn to make her baby look beautiful and protect her from evil eyes.

Discussion

As a critical milestone in the life of newborns, postnatal care is an important component of newborn survival. The study revealed an important link between neonatal deaths and postnatal practices such as skin-to-skin care, early initiation of breastfeeding, and home visits by health workers. The analysis shows that caregivers had only a moderate amount of knowledge of newborn care practices and that this gap in knowledge was due to a combination of deep-rooted socio-cultural practices, lack of health knowledge, and economic barriers. The socioeconomic situation of the women determined whether or not they made institutional visits for postnatal care, whereas the differences did not manifest themselves in the home visits by community workers. A major challenge to effective postnatal care in Bihar is that over one-fifth of deliveries still happen outside the formal system. The barriers to the use of PNC are mainly concentrated among these deliveries. This further reinforces the significance of facility delivery considering that it is indeed a gateway to good postnatal health behaviours.

The use of postnatal services is mainly limited due to the low perceived value of postnatal visits and the lack of awareness. This is linked to inadequate counselling at the facilities, shorter hospital stays, misconceptions, and inadequate community-based interventions. All this even though the Bihar government has launched cost-effective interventions to reduce newborn deaths caused by the lack of postnatal care. Community-based interventions were found to be effective in shaping the socio-cultural practices related to postnatal care in the study area. The role of frontline workers is critical as, through interpersonal communication and culturally contextualised messages, they bring about a behavioural change in the adoption of healthy postnatal practices. Interventions aimed at changing the behaviour of families towards newborn care practices, however, are few. The gap in service delivery was quite pronounced, with home visits by ASHA workers being limited to once after birth and with almost a third of the target population remaining untouched by these community workers. As all countries aim to achieve SDG-3.2, there is a compelling rationale for strengthening the community linkages and enhancing the postnatal home visits by health workers in accordance with the guidelines.

References

Bang, A. T., Bang, R. A., Baitule, S. B., Reddy, M. H., & Deshmukh, M. D. (1999). Effect of home-based neonatal care and management of sepsis on neonatal mortality: field trial in rural India. *The Lancet*, *354*(9194), 1955–1961.

Chaturvedi, M., Nandan, D., & Gupta, S. C. (2007). Rapid assessment of infant-feeding practices in Agra district. *Indian Journal of Community Medicine*, *32*(3), 227.

Chellaiyan, V. G., Liaquathali, F., & Marudupandiyan, J. (2020). Healthy nutrition for a healthy child: A review on infant feeding in India. *Journal of Family & Community Medicine*, *27*(1), 1.

Georgieff, M., Piovanetti, Y., & Queenan, J. (1997). Breastfeeding and the use of human milk. *Pediatrics*, 100(6), 1035–1039. https://doi.org/10.1542/peds.100.6.1035
Godhia, M. L., & Patel, N. (2013). Colostrum—its Composition, Benefits as a Nutraceutical—A Review. *Current Research in Nutrition and Food Science Journal*, *1*(1), 37–47.
Home Based Newborn Care, Operational Guildelines (2011). Published by Ministry of Health and Family Welfare, GoI.
Jones, G., Steketee, R. W., Black, R. E., Bhutta, Z. A., Morris, S. S., & Bellagio Child Survival Study Group. (2003). How many child deaths can we prevent this year?. *The Lancet*, *362*(9377), 65–71.
Kumar, V., Mohanty, S., Kumar, A., Misra, R. P., Santosham, M., Awasthi, S., … Saksham Study Group. (2008). Effect of community-based behaviour change management on neonatal mortality in Shivgarh, Uttar Pradesh, India: a cluster-randomised controlled trial. *The Lancet*, *372*(9644), 1151–1162.
Kyomuhendo, G. B. (2003). Low use of rural maternity services in Uganda: impact of women's status, traditional beliefs and limited resources. *Reproductive Health Matters*, *11*(21), 16–26.
Lawn, J., & Kerber, K. (2006). *Opportunities for Africa's Newborns: Practical data, policy and programmatic support for newborn care in Africa*. Partnership for Maternal, Newborn and Child Health, Cape Town, 32.
MacArthur, C., Winter, H. R., Bick, D. E., Knowles, H., Lilford, R., Henderson, C., … Gee, H. (2002). Effects of redesigned community postnatal care on women's health 4 months after birth: a cluster randomised controlled trial. *The Lancet*, *359*(9304), 378–385.
Mandal, P. K., Sardar, J. C., Chatterjee, C., Lahiri, S. K., & Ghosh, P. K. (2007). A study on breast feeding practices among infants in a rural area of west Bengal. *Indian J Prev Soc Med*, *38*(1–2), 28–31.
Moore, E. R., Bergman, N., Anderson, G. C., & Medley, N. (2016). Early skin-to-skin contact for mothers and their healthy newborn infants. *Cochrane Database of Systematic Reviews*, (11).
Mullany, L. C., Katz, J., Li, Y. M., Khatry, S. K., LeClerq, S. C., Darmstadt, G. L., & Tielsch, J. M. (2008). Breast-feeding patterns, time to initiation, and mortality risk among newborns in southern Nepal. *The Journal of Nutrition*, *138*(3), 599–603.
Mukherjee, K., & Venugopal, P. N. (2018). Colostrum avoidance and breastfeeding practices among mothers of Khos tribal Community of Uttarakhand: a community-based cross-sectional study. *Journal of the Anthropological Survey of India*, *67*(1), 45–55.
Pathi, S. (2005). Breast feeding practices in a rural ICDS block of Khallikote. *South Orissa Indian J Community Med*, *30*, 10–2.

Probandari, A., Arcita, A., Kothijah, K., & Pamungkasari, E. P. (2017). Barriers to utilization of postnatal care at village level in Klaten district, central Java Province, Indonesia. *BMC Health Services Research, 17*(1), 1–9.

Raven, J. H., Chen, Q., Tolhurst, R. J., & Garner, P. (2007). Traditional beliefs and practices in the postpartum period in Fujian Province, China: a qualitative study. *BMC Pregnancy and Childbirth, 7*(1), 1–11.

Randhawa, A., Chaudhary, N., Gill, B. S., Singh, A., Garg, V., & Balgir, R. S. (2019). A population-based cross-sectional study to determine the practices of breastfeeding among the lactating mothers of Patiala city. *Journal of Family Medicine and Primary Care*, 8(10), 3207–3213. https://doi.org/10.4103/jfmpc.jfmpc_549_19

Singh, A., Padmadas, S. S., Mishra, U. S., Pallikadavath, S., Johnson, F. A., & Matthews, Z. (2012). Socio-Economic Inequalities in the Use of Postnatal Care in India. *PLoS ONE, 7*(5), e37037. https://doi.org/10.1371/journal.pone.0037037

UNICEF (2016). *From the first hour of life: making the case for improved infant and young child feeding everywhere*. New York.

WHO (1998), *Postpartum care of the mother and newborn: a practical guide.* WHO: Geneva

WHO. (2014). *Every newborn: an action plan to end preventable deaths.* Geneva: World Health Organization.

CHAPTER 7

Access to Sick Newborn Care Services: Efficiency, Adequacy, and Equity

Introduction

A well-developed health system is crucial for improving the health outcomes of a population. Currently, India is far from achieving the SDG target of reducing neonatal deaths to 12 per 1000 live births; as per NFHS-4 estimates, it is on an average 2.4 times higher than the target laid down in the SDGs. Achieving the SDG targets requires care for every newborn, which includes the most vulnerable—the small and the sick. A critical step in overcoming the barriers to newborn survival is to extend the care facilities to all the newborns, particularly the sick ones. The expansion of healthcare facilities to sick newborns is highly desirable because they are at a higher risk of death and require intensive inpatient care. Health infrastructure, its availability, and its quality—as discussed in Chaps. 3 and 5—are critical to newborn survival. Poor availability of clinical services and low quality of care has been recognised as one of the most common bottlenecks to MNH services in India (Dickson et al. 2014; Bhutta et al. 2014).

The Indian government launched the National Rural Health Mission in 2005 to reinforce and ensure an adequate and equitable supply of health infrastructure. With the launch of NRHM, the focus on newborn care became central to the government's child health strategies. Facility Based Newborn Care (FBNC) programme is one of the key initiatives launched by the Ministry of Health & Family Welfare, Government of India

S. R. Mahapatro, *Towards Newborn Survival*,
https://doi.org/10.1007/978-981-19-3417-9_7

(MoHFW, GoI) under NRHM and the RMNCH+A strategic programme to improve the survival chances and health status of newborn. Under this programme, Newborn Care Corners (NBCCs), Newborn Stabilization Units (NBSUs), and Special Newborn Care Units (SNCUs) are being established at different levels of healthcare facilities (Two year progress of SNCUs in India, 2011–12 & 2012–13). This has led to a nationwide creation of Newborn Care Corners (NBCCs) at every point of childbirth. Newborn Stabilization Units (NBSUs) are established at CHCs or at First Referral Units (FRUs), while sick/special newborn care units (SNCUs) are established at district hospitals (Neogi et al. 2016).

Historically, the care of small and sick newborn babies has always been executed at the secondary or tertiary care units situated in the hospitals (e.g. neonatal intensive care units). In India, facility care for newborns began in the early 1960s in a few teaching hospitals. Over time, emphasis was given on providing essential newborn services at home as well. For this, the National Neonatology Forum (NNF) established accreditation norms for quality newborn care at health facilities. FBNC became functional in 1994 in 26 districts with the strengthening of district and sub-district health facilities mainly through the provision of equipment (radiant warmers, resuscitation equipment, weighing scales, and phototherapy units) and training and through oversight (www.jhpiego.org 2013). Sick newborns, who are identified with signs of danger and complicated deliveries assisted by health workers, are referred to intensive care. Programmers and policy makers have observed that facility-based newborn care corners, specifically SNCU interventions, have played a dramatic role in improving newborn survival and providing the newborns a healthy life eventually.

The concept of SNCU is based on the lessons learnt from the 'Purulia Model'. Purulia was one of the backward districts of West Bengal, with a high burden of neonatal mortality. With the establishment of SNCUs in the district in 2003, it was observed that, compared with the baseline, neonatal mortality fell by 14 per cent in the first year and by 21 per cent in the second year. The success of this model has driven its replication across the nation as evident from the central government's initiative to start SNCUs in 6000 districts of the country under NRHM. Sick/special newborn care units are established at district hospitals with an annual delivery load of more than 3000 to provide for sick newborns. An SNCU is a separate unit with proximity to the labour room, managed by adequately trained doctors, staff nurses, and support staff to provide 24/7 services. Availability of life-saving interventions, such as ventilators, oxygen, essential technologies, uninterrupted water and electricity, and proper medication increase the survival of sick newborns.

The Empowered Action Group states of India consistently lag behind the other states in providing quality services due to the shortage of an adequate health infrastructure. The shortage of SNCU facilities is also visible in these states. The data presented in Table 7.1 shows the availability of SNCUs, NBSUs, and NBCCs in these states. The distribution of neonatal mortality across the states of India shows a skewed pattern whereby the districts of some states have already achieved the SDG targets, while a majority of the districts in the less-developed states continue to have high NMR. In this context, an active role of the state is deemed to be critical for introducing effective strategies to address the socio-cultural and structural barriers to newborn survival. In Bihar, SNCUs started operating in 2008 with technical support from the UNICEF and the National Neonatology Forum. Currently, 43 SNCUs have been set up across the state. Neonates born with complications are generally recommended for admission in newborn care corners. Hence, the admission mostly occurs in the early neonatal period. As per NHM (2020), the proportion of early neonatal deaths to infant deaths is the highest in Bihar among all the EAG states, indicating the need for proper and adequate attention during the early neonatal period. Since the number of children born is high in Bihar, there is, naturally, a high demand for newborn care corners too. The

Table 7.1 Neonatal deaths and newborn care facilities across EAG states, 2020

EAG states	*Neonatal mortality*	*Early NMR*	*Proportion of early neonatal deaths to infant deaths*	*SNCU*	*NBSU*	*NBCC*
Bihar	25	20	61.8	43	41	708
Chhattisgarh	29	22	54.5	23	134	1249
Jharkhand	21	17	56.5	19	27	594
Madhya Pradesh	35	26	52.8	54	62	1303
Odisha	31	24	59.9	40	45	730
Rajasthan	26	20	54.2	59	286	2065
Uttar Pradesh	32	24	56.4	82	237	1820
Uttarakhand	22	17	55.6	5	47	129

Source: National Health Mission (2020)

number of NBCCs and NBSUs, however, is relatively lower in Bihar than in states like Chhattisgarh, Madhya Pradesh, Uttar Pradesh, and Rajasthan. This implies that there is a need to invest more towards increasing the size and functionality of sick newborn care units. Besides the adequacy of SNCUs, their functionality and quality are important too for analysing and understanding newborn survival. As per Bihar PIP (2013–2014), 484 NBCCs were approved and made operational. However, of the approved 40 NBSUs and 39 SNCUs, only one-fifth are operational. This reflects that, although in terms of numbers, there has been an increase in newborn care units, it is equally important for them to be functioning and providing quality care from the perspective of newborn health.

The following section of the chapter discusses the details of SNCUs, including their quality and functioning.

Admission in SNCU: Profile and Outcomes

The status of newborn health underscores the weaknesses of the public health system of a state. Table 7.2 presents district-wise information on SNCU admission, deaths, and facilities as available in the SNCU online database of the National Health Mission (2020). Among the surveyed districts, Rohtas (20 per cent), followed by West Champaran (15 per cent), recorded the highest number of newborn deaths. Substantial gender differences in admission, with the proportion of male newborns exceeding that of female newborns, were observed. In the district of West Champaran, the difference was minimal, with 47 per cent of all admissions being those of female newborns. The newborns admitted in SNCUs were mainly outborns referred by a health facility. However, in Khagaria (71 per cent), followed by Kishanganj (59 per cent), inborn admissions were more than half of the total admissions. In Madhubani, the health workers had referred most of the cases to an SNCU. Households arranged for their own transportation to an SNCU centre most of the time. Only in Nalanda more than 70 per cent SNCU admissions were done through government-provided transport. Nalanda also had the maximum number of low-weight babies admitted in SNCU. The progress of SNCUs, especially in numbers, has been increasing over time in the state. Bihar had 10 SNCUs in 2013, with 50 per cent of them having 12 beds. By 2018, the government had set up 43 SNCUs.

As per the guidelines, each SNCU has to have 12 beds and, at least, 1 doctor supported by an adequate number of paramedical staff. In the

Table 7.2 District-wise SNCU deaths, newborn admission, and healthcare resources

District	*Jehanabad*	*Nalanda*	*Rohtas*	*Kishanganj*	*Madhubani*	*Muzaffarpur*	*Khagaria*	*West Champaran*
Percentage deaths	5.1	6.8	20.1	8.0	6.4	6.8	8.1	15.2
Male newborns admitted	62.6	60.5	58.2	59.9	63.4	63.0	59.5	52.8
Govt. provided	29.9	70.7	37.1	23.4	7.0	62.6	21.3	31.7
Inborn	33.0	38.9	30.2	59.1	36.6	23.9	71.4	30.5
Outborn (community-referred)	5.0	6.0	19.3	0.3	39.2	5.2	9.2	30.0
Outborn (health facility referred)	62.0	55.2	50.5	40.6	24.3	71.1	19.4	39.6
<1500 gm	7.6	12.4	11.1	8.0	8.0	12.7	10.0	6.9
>37 week	87.4	1.2	74.1	0.0	71.9	33.2	12.5	43.2
Hospital beds	12	13	11	11	16	12	13	12
Doctors	5	4	3	2	1	2	2	6
Nurses	13	9	11	1	10	8	8	3

Source: www.sncuindiaonline.org

study districts, Rohtas and Kishanganj were found to be lacking the number of beds required as per the guidelines. The shortage of nursing staff was the highest in Kishanganj and West Champaran, while Madhubani had only one doctor per SNCU.

Most of the existing information available with governments is about the profile of a newborn at the time of admission and the physical resources available. The setting up of SNCUs is not enough on its own. Their functioning, quality, and accessibility matter too, which, however, is not captured in the existing data. Since SNCUs play a key role in saving newborn lives, it is essential to monitor their functioning to ensure that the newborn care services are provided effectively. The high risk of neonatal mortality and the dearth of research in this area prompt an exploration of issues related to the quality of SNCU care and the constraining factors. The following section analyses these aspects through the household survey.

The data collected on SNCUs in the survey pertained to admission in both private and public facilities (Table 7.3). The study data confirmed the significance of SNCU admission to increasing the newborn survival. In the surveyed districts, 11 per cent mothers reported that their newborns had signs of difficulty during the neonatal period. Nearly 95 per cent of them went to a doctor, and almost half of them were recommended to go for specialised newborn care. Overall, 5 per cent of the newborns were admitted in newborn care corners at secondary and tertiary levels. Newborns delivered in facilities had higher chances of SNCU admission (6 per cent) than those who were delivered at home (3 per cent). Admission in SNCU occurred through in-facility transfer or referrals by community workers. A gender differential in SNCU admission was observed, with a higher proportion of male (64.4 per cent) over female newborns (35.6 per cent) being admitted to SNCUs. The proportion of SNCU deaths to total neonatal deaths was 42 per cent; it was higher among inborns (43 per cent) than outborns (39 per cent), and the case-fatality rate was 0.9 per cent of the sample. Almost half of the newborns were admitted within a day (47 per cent), and over a third of those who were admitted (34 per cent) stayed for more than seven days. In rural India, the family of a newborn opts for SNCU treatment at the last minute when all home remedies and informal care measures have failed, which only increases the complications. Identifying difficult signs in time and reaching out for medical care is crucial, therefore.

Table 7.3 Admission in sick newborn care units and details of stay

Admission in SNCU and details of stay	*Percentage*
SNCU admission & neonatal survival	7.9***(p<0.005)
Babies admitted in SNCU (N=117)	5.1
SNCU admission by place of delivery	
Home	3
Facility	6
Gender	
Male	64.4
Female	35.6
SNCU survival	82
SNCU deaths to total deaths (N=51)	41.6
Timing of admission in SNCU	
Within 24 hours	47.2
After 24 hours	52.8
Duration in SNCU	
0–7 days	66
More than seven days	34
Average number of days stayed	7
Level of care referred	
Level 1 NSU	15.7
Level 2 SNCU	77.9
Level 3 NICU	6.4
Reason of death (N = 21)	
LBW/premature	35.8
Birth asphyxia	44.1
Jaundice	10.1
Infection/congenital malformation	10
District-wise deaths	
Rohtas	13.4
Kishanganj	14.1
Madhubani	16.6
Muzaffarpur	16.6
West Champaran	18.2
Jehanabad	19.8
Khagaria	26.7
Nalanda	36.1
SNCU expenditure (total)	15,084
SNCU expenditure (public)	987

Source: Field data

The survey data reveals that a majority (78 per cent) of the neonates admitted in an SNCU were referred to level II care (requiring ventilation) and 16 per cent to level I care. The major cause of death in an SNCU was birth asphyxia (44 per cent), followed by prematurity/low birth weight (36 per cent). Jaundice and other illnesses respectively accounted for 10 per cent of total SNCU deaths. Our results corroborate the findings of the other studies that have found prematurity, followed by birth asphyxia and infection, as the leading cause of death (Kumar et al. 2019) among newborns. According to one study, severe hypothermia, respiratory distress, admission within the first 24 hours of life, absence of health personnel during transport, and referral from a hospital had significant correlation with mortality (Aggarwal et al. 2015).

Our analysis showed that of the total admissions, the survival rate or successful discharge was 82 per cent, mainly because of timely arrival and appropriate care. However, geographical variations in neonatal deaths were observed across the districts. The proportion of SNCU deaths was the highest in Nalanda (36 per cent), followed by Khagaria (27 per cent). Low birth weight and gestational age less than 37 weeks perhaps reduced the survival benefits in these districts as described in Table 7.2. On the other hand, Rohtas (13.4 per cent) and Kishanganj (14 per cent) recorded the lowest proportion of deaths. Timely access to and quality of care in an SNCU were important contributing factors to neonatal survival, apart from the health status of the baby at the time of admission.

Cost of SNCU Services

Access to quality and affordable healthcare for neonates is important to achieve the SDG targets on NMR. As facility birth is increasing, the demand for sick newborn care is also increasing gradually. An estimate by Prinja et al. (2013) on the cost of providing SNCU care in India showed that per capita neonate treatment and per bed-day treatment cost the government Rs. 4581 (USD 102) and Rs. 818 (USD 18.2) respectively. In the absence of adequate care at public facilities, most admissions take place at private facilities, resulting in high out-of-pocket expenditure for households. The average cost of treatment in an SNCU (public and private) was Rs. 15,084, while the OOPE was around Rs. 1000 among those who went to government-supported SNCUs.

The average expenditure estimated during the stay in an SNCU was proportional to the number of deaths reported in the respective districts. The districts of Khagaria (Rs. 23,825) and West Champaran (Rs. 23,777) had the highest expenditure on SNCU. Both had high neonatal deaths of 3.2 per cent and 3.7 per cent, out of which 26.7 per cent and 18.9 per cent deaths respectively were of neonates who required admission to an

SNCU. The lowest average expenses were observed in Kishanganj (Rs. 1912), where, out of the 2.7 per cent total neonatal deaths, 14.1 per cent were of those who required SNCU care. At 36.1 per cent, Nalanda had the highest proportion of SNCU admissions and 2.4 per cent of total neonatal deaths. The expenses made on neonatal care in an SNCU, however, depended on the criticality of the illness and the availability of the facilities. High cost of SNCU services, as observed from the field, was one of the major impediments to access to healthcare for the newborn.

Neonatal Deaths and Quality of Care at SNCU

Among the SNCU admissions, 38 per cent mothers reported encountering difficulties at the centre. Among the difficulties cited, high cost of SNCU care was reported by almost three-quarters of the respondents (74 per cent). The other difficulties were long waiting time (22.7 per cent), lack of infrastructure/staff (7.2 per cent), and improper staff behaviour (4.8 per cent). The respondents were asked about their perception of the quality of services received, and the responses were recorded as very good, good, bad, and very bad. 'Very bad' and 'bad' responses were coded as poor quality of services, and 'good' and 'very good' responses were coded as better quality. A composite index of quality of care was computed, consisting of six indices of quality of care such as cost, waiting time, staff behaviour, availability of drugs, and any other challenges. The SNCU quality of care index (SQCI) showed that almost three-quarters of the respondents, who had admitted their babies to an SNCU, reported the quality of care as better. A clear association of the quality of services with neonatal survival was observed as poor quality of care coincided with a higher number of deaths. In the study, the incidence of newborn deaths was 27 per 1000 live births among those experienced poor quality of care, whereas it declined to 15 per 1000 live births among those who reported having received better quality of care (Table 7.4).

> *I had a normal delivery in a public health facility; a male baby was born weighing 3100gm. The birth place was hygienic, and the delivery was safely done. After the delivery, however, the baby did not cry and showed signs of laziness. After consulting the doctor, we admitted the baby to level II (ventilation) of SNCU within 24 hours and kept him in the SNCU for eight days, but he could not survive.* (Manti Devi, Nalanda district)

Table 7.4 Quality of care at SNCU

Difficulties at SNCU (N = 45)	*38.1*
High cost	74.1
Lack of infrastructure/staff	7.2
Long waiting time	22.7
Staff behaviour not good	4.8
Drugs not available	0
Other	7.6
Quality of services (perceived experience)	
Very bad	11.4
Bad	14.8
Good	71.1
Very good	2.7
Poor SQCI & neonatal death	26.7
Better SQCI & neonatal death	15
Infrastructure in newborn corner	
24-hour running water	91.4
Elbow-operated wash machine	76.5
Soap availability	80.5
Hand wash	80.5
Wearing gowns	88.5
Wearing sleepers	77.1
Wearing mask and caps	85.7

Source: Field data

She reported that her family had to bear a disproportionate burden of expenditure for the stay at the SNCU and that the quality of care provided was also not satisfactory.

> *A respondent who admitted her baby in a private SNCU described her experience: There were complications in child birth; the baby was struggling to breathe. There was a delay in delivery, and the baby ingested some of the meconium. The baby was kept in the SNCU for a month and we spent three lakh rupees, but she could not survive due to reduced supply of blood and oxygen to the brain.*

Health infrastructure is an important indicator for improving the health outcomes and for the healthcare policy of a country (Ghosh and Dinda 2017). It is also an indicator of the basic support for the delivery of health services. It is well established that the presence of trained health professionals at well-equipped health centres helps increase health-seeking behaviour. As part of this study, an assessment of the facilities in the villages/urban areas was carried out to ascertain the capacity of the health facilities. The availability and quality of services, equipment, labour rooms, operation theatre, newborn corners, drug stores, maternity wards, labs, SNCUs, oxygen cylinders, ACs, stabilisers, and so on was assessed. Information on infrastructure and equipment was gathered through interviews with medical officers in-charge (MOIC) at the PHCs, hospital managers at the DHs, and staff nurses as well as through direct observation. The assessment of SNCU facilities showed that around 80 per cent of newborn care centres had the running water facility, elbow-operated wash machines, and medical shops and health personnel who wore gowns, sleepers, and masks while holding a baby or taking care of it.

Barriers to SNCU Care

In the previous section, we had discussed the performance of SNCU and the pattern of admission in the study districts. The next section explains the difficulties experienced in SNCU facilities and the bottlenecks of admission to SNCUs.

Gender Discrimination

Despite biological advantages, early neonatal mortality was higher among girls in the study and the plausible reason is the gender disparate in SNCU admission. Of the total sick newborns admitted to SNCUs, males (65 per cent) vastly outnumbered females (35 per cent). While 96 per cent male newborns with signs of danger went to a doctor, 86 per cent of females did so. Other studies too have shown that male admissions in newborn care centres are higher than female admissions (MoHFW 2013) and that more female infants die compared with male infants following post-delivery discharge from a healthcare facility (Malhotra et al. 2012). The higher number of deaths among female newborn is the reflection of differential care-seeking behaviour that is embedded in the deep-rooted cultural preferences for sons over daughters. The present study revealed gender differences in postnatal check-ups too, with 56 per cent male newborns, compared to 52 per cent female newborns, taken for check-ups. The data revealed a significant gender difference in health expenditure on postnatal visits and SNCU care. For a male child, on an average, an amount of Rs. 1506 was spent on a PNC visit and almost Rs. 20,000 on treatment (Rs.

19,620) in a newborn centre. Among female newborns, the corresponding expenditure was five times (Rs. 276) and four times (Rs. 4556) lower. This is evidence that the cultural bias towards sons creates gender inequality in postnatal visits and SNCU care.

Poverty and High Out-of-Pocket Expenses

Cost of care, as a major difficulty in accessing SNCU services, was reported by almost three-quarters of the respondents. Longer duration of stay for the critically ill newborns, compounded by higher per-day treatment, increased the cost of services. The survey found that, on an average, a family spent Rs. 15000 on SNCU care (public as well as private facilities) and that the OOPE on SNCU in public facilities was Rs. 1000. The SNCU expenditure among the poorest was seven times their monthly expenditure, whereas for the richest, the ratio of SNCU expenditure to monthly expenditure was 0.81. The disproportionate expenditure burden among the lower class reinforces class inequality and keeps many vulnerable newborns from poor families deprived of SNCU care despite the pressing need for medical attention.

A woman from Khagaria, who had given birth to low birth weight twins, recalled:

> *The OOPE on SNCU care put a major financial burden on my family. The male child weighed 1400 gms and the female child 1500 gms. The baby girl was in a very critical condition at birth. She was taken to a private hospital after 48 hours, and admitted in ICU. She was hospitalised for five days, but when her condition did not improve, she was referred to PMCH, Patna. Due to poverty, we had to sell two katthas of land, which gave us two lakh rupees for the baby's treatment. When we ran out money, we brought the baby back home, where she passed away 24 hours later.*

Such stories explain not only the financial but also the psychological and emotional challenges the poor households face for the survival of their babies.

Socioeconomic Inequity in SNCU Service Utilisation

It has become well understood from the earlier chapters that poor and lower-caste women had less access to healthcare services. Given the multi-layered nature of Bihar's society, with the existence of multiple socioeconomic groups, it is important to look not only at inter-class but also at the intra-class variations in healthcare access. We found that low-income status, intersecting with poor social status, lowered the utilisation of SNCU services. In this connection, studies have found that although socioeconomic inequalities in neonatal mortality are declining, babies born into wealthier households with a high educational level have a substantial survival advantage (McKinnon et al. 2014).

In the study it was found that lower-caste and lower-class women made fewer SNCU visits (4 per cent) compared to women of lower class of non-SC/ST castes (6.1 per cent). Similarly, SC/ST women with no education were less likely to visit SNCU facilities (3.1 per cent) than non-SC/ST women with no education (5.3 per cent). The SNCU expenditure was seven times the monthly expenditure among the poorest, whereas for the richest, the ratio of SNCU expenditure to monthly expenditure was 0.81. This signifies that the economic condition of a family is critical in deciding admission to an SNCU. In high-focused states of India, the risk of under-five mortality among the affluent as well as the deprived castes has declined after the introduction of NRHM. Despite this, children belonging to SC/ST experience a higher mortality than children of non-SC/ST castes, and this caste-based gap is majorly due to the educational differential (Bora et al. 2019). The caste identity appears to interact with other social determinants in creating inequality in accessing SNCU services. The socioeconomic differences in SNCU visits in the survey demonstrate that caste, class, education of mother, and gender of baby determine access to SNCU care, and the inequalities in healthcare expenditure are more pronounced among the poor than the rich.

Discussion

Bihar has witnessed a reduction in neonatal mortality after a long gap, though the NMR of the state is higher than that of many states and the all-India average. The expansion in the SNCU services appears to have played a critical role in this. Research pertaining to the availability of SNCU care and the barriers to access to the services is relatively scant in India, including Bihar. I took this opportunity to have a detailed understanding of the SNCU services in Bihar and the factors impeding access to SNCU care through a household survey. The detailed investigation into morbidity, expenditure, and quality of care made in the survey may help programmers and policy makers in modifying the treatment and intervention plans.

The study showed that eight out of ten newborns survived after being admitted to an SNCU, reflecting the significance of newborn care units in the survival of sick newborns. The SQCI showed that newborns with an access to better quality care had higher chances of survival than those who received low quality of services, which emphasises the need to improve the quality of services. Birth asphyxia, followed by prematurity/low birth weight, was the leading cause of SNCU admission as well as death. Sluggish health infrastructure, lack of awareness, gender discrimination, and higher financial burden were the most prevalent impeding factors for SNCU admission and hence newborn survival. The analysis drawn from the chapter shows that the market forces increase the cost of services, burden of OOPE among the poor, and obstruct the access to affordable SNCU care. This pushes many families into the poverty trap and widens the class inequalities. The rigid social norms create significant gender differences in newborn care as reflected in postnatal visits, SNCU admissions, and postnatal expenses. While each social determinant has its own significance, the intersection of such determinants reveals newborns from deprived communities have less access to SNCU care. This indicates the need for strategies in an intersectional approach for the inclusion of the marginalised.

The findings of the study also underscore the need for specialised newborn care to be provided at a low cost with improved quality. Promoting early referral and community-facility linkage and combating gender bias in newborn care are thus critical. To help families, especially the poor ones, to cope up with high SNCU costs, it is desirable to implement cost-effective interventions and include newborns in insurance programmes. Ensuring equitable and affordable intensive care to sick newborns of all socioeconomic strata is pivotal for reducing neonatal mortality.

References

Aggarwal, K. C., Gupta, R., Sharma, S., Sehgal, R., & Roy, M. P. (2015). Mortality in newborns referred to tertiary hospital: An introspection. *Journal of Family Medicine and Primary Care*, 4(3), 435.

Bhutta, Z. A., Das, J. K., Bahl, R., Lawn, J. E., Salam, R. A., Paul, V. K., ... & Lancet Every Newborn Study Group. (2014). Can available interventions end preventable deaths in mothers, newborn babies, and stillbirths, and at what cost?. *The Lancet*, 384(9940), 347–370.

Bora, J. K., Raushan, R., & Lutz, W. (2019). The persistent influence of caste on under-five mortality: Factors that explain the caste-based gap in high focus Indian states. *Plos One*, 14(8), e0211086.

Dickson, K. E., Simen-Kapeu, A., Kinney, M. V., Huicho, L., Vesel, L., Lackritz, E., & Lancet Every Newborn Study Group. (2014). Every Newborn: health-systems bottlenecks and strategies to accelerate scale-up in countries. *The Lancet*, 384(9941), 438–454.

https://nhm.gov.in/images/pdf/programmes/child-health/annual-report/Two_Year_Progress_of_SNCUs-A_Brief_Report_(2011-12_&_2012-13).pdf

Ghosh, D. & Dinda, S. (2017). *Health infrastructure and economic development in India*. IGI Global https://doi.org/10.4018/978-1-5225-3168-5.ch005

Kumar, R., Mundhra, J. A., Jain, S., & Jain, S. (2019). Morbidity and mortality profile of neonates admitted in special newborn care unit of a teaching hospital in Uttarakhand, India. *Int J Res Med Sci*, 7(1), 241–246.

Malhotra, S., Neogi, S. B., Raj, S. S., Sharma, K., & Zodpey, S. P. (2012). Tracking survival of institutional births for neonatal period-feasibility at district hospitals. *Indian Pediatrics*, 49(6), 479–480.

McKinnon, B., Harper, S., Kaufman, J. S., & Bergevin, Y. (2014). Socioeconomic inequality in neonatal mortality in countries of low and middle income: a multicountry analysis. *The Lancet Global Health*, 2(3), e165–e173.

Ministry of Health and Family Welfare, Government of India (2013). Child Health Division, Two year progress report of special newborn care units in India.

Neogi, S. B., Khanna, R., Chauhan, M., Sharma, J., Gupta, G., Srivastava, R., … Paul, V. K. (2016). Inpatient care of small and sick newborns in healthcare facilities. *Journal of Perinatology*, 36(3), S18–S23.

Prinja, S., Manchanda, N., Mohan, P., Gupta, G., Sethy, G., Sen, A., ... Kumar, R. (2013). Cost of neonatal intensive care delivered through district level public hospitals in India. *Indian Pediatrics*, 50(9), 839–846.

Two year progress of SNCUs in India, A Brief Report, 2011–12 & 2012–13 published by Child Health Division, Ministry of Health and Family Welfare, Government of India. https://nhm.gov.in/images/pdf/programmes/child-health/annual-report/Two_Year_Progress_of_SNCUs-A_Brief_Report_(2011-12_&_2012-13).pdf

CHAPTER 8

Direct Benefit Transfer and Newborn Health

Introduction

Reducing preventable newborn deaths through various interventions is the established developmental approach taken by governments across the globe. Poor and marginalised women face multiple demand- and supply-side constraints in accessing public health services. While supply-side barriers are addressed through revamping the health system such as improvement in quality-of-service delivery, investment in health infrastructure, and increasing budgetary allocation, overcoming the demand-side barriers requires various pro-poor public policies and behavioural change interventions. Many developing countries, including India, have designed a variety of demand-side interventions for maternal and child survival. There are two main policy approaches to increasing the demand for maternal and newborn health services under these interventions. One is to change the health-seeking behaviour through community-based interventions such as community-based education or by disseminating information through participatory women's groups (Hurst et al. 2015). The other approach is to provide financial incentives (like cash transfers and vouchers) for public facility delivery. Such pro-poor public policies and their linkages with MNH outcomes in a poor socioeconomic context have profound implications on political economy of the health sector. The previous chapters of the book underscored the importance of community-level interventions in relation to newborn health. This chapter provides a

S. R. Mahapatro, *Towards Newborn Survival*,
https://doi.org/10.1007/978-981-19-3417-9_8

critical assessment of Direct Benefit Transfer[1] (DBT) in removing financial barriers that impede the use of MCH services and explores the implementation challenges of such programmes.

The survival and well-being of newborn babies is positively allied with the use of institutional care along the continuum from pregnancy to the postnatal period. Seeking institutional care in resource-poor regions, however, is challenging, particularly for the poor and marginalised. Evidence shows that healthcare is largely financed by households and lack of capacity to pay due to high OOPE remains a major barrier to healthcare needs (Borooah 2010). Studies from Asia and sub-Saharan Africa (SSA) estimate that maternal healthcare cost accounts for 1–5 per cent of total annual household expenditure and can increase to 5–34 per cent if complications occur (Brearley et al. 2012). Informal payments for maternity services, arrangements for transportation and accommodation, cost of medicines, and so on increase the cost of delivery of and care for the newborn (Borooah 2010; Pathak et al. 2010). Financial constraints can cause delays or an avoidance for care, increasing the health complications among the newborn and the mothers, which can further escalate the cost of care and push a household into the poverty trap.

The Indian government, since the 1990s, has initiated a series of programmes to increase the use of MNCH services. The government launched the Child Survival and Safe Motherhood (CSSM) programme for 1992–1997; however, the programme failed to increase the number of birth facilities. Subsequently, the reproductive and child health (RCH I) programme (1997–2004) and RCH II (2005) were initiated under CSSM to strengthen referral units for childbirth and promote institutional delivery (Huque et al. 1996). In 2005, major reforms were made in the health sector with the setting up of NRHM. The post-NRHM period witnessed major developments in policies and programmes that impacted use of MNH services and government has infused substantial resources for improving the health outcomes. Various pro-poor programmes such as JSY, JSSK, and PMMVY were implemented within the larger institutional framework of the National Health Mission (NHM) for upscaling the use of maternal and child health services and reducing economic burden of families. Transfer of cash incentives under these schemes is considered as the most promising approach to increase facility delivery, empower women

[1]The term DBT is used interchangeably with financial interventions or the conditional cash transfer (CCT) scheme in the chapter.

to access institutional care (Gaarder et al. 2010), and ameliorate persistent problems of OOPE.

Janani Suraksha Yojana (JSY) is the world's largest centrally funded conditional cash transfer (CCT) programme (Lim et al. 2010). The scheme incentivises women for deliveries in public health facilities with the goal of improving maternal and newborn survival. The scheme was launched in 18 high-focused states (having poor MCH indicators) and 10 low-focused states. By 2018–2019, more than one-crore beneficiaries were getting covered under the scheme, with an estimated budget allocation of Rs. 19.8 billion. In the high-focused states, women delivering at a public facility are offered a sum of Rs. 1400 or $19.3 in rural areas (US $1 = 72.26) and a sum of Rs. 1000 or $ 13.7 in urban areas. In low-focused states, women are eligible to receive Rs. 700 or $9.6 in rural areas and Rs. 600 or $8.2 in urban areas. The cash payment is offered to all women in high-focused states; by contrast, only women belonging to below poverty line households, those from marginalised communities, and those with up to two children are given the incentive in low-focused states. Following JSY, the Janani Shishu Suraksha Karyakram (JSSK) was launched in 2011 to further reduce out-of-pocket expenditure through free drugs, diet, and diagnosis of sick newborn for up to one year. Undernutrition among pregnant women is one of the major challenges in India that affects newborn health and prevails mostly among the low economic class. Owing to economic difficulties, women from the low economic strata engage in paid work till the last stage of pregnancy and resume work soon after childbirth. Continued employment, without a sufficient gap during pregnancy and the postpartum period, affects the health of the mother as well as the newborn. To address such issues, the Pradhan Mantri Matru Vandana Yojana (PMMVY) was implemented in 2017 across India in accordance with the National Food Security Act, 2013 with an increase in the size of cash benefits. Under PMMVY, a sum of Rs. 5000 or $68.8 is provided for the first live birth. The remaining cash incentive of Rs. 1000 is given as per the approved norms of JSY, so that women get, on an average, Rs. 6000 or $82.5 for the first live birth. The women receive the benefit in three instalments: First, after registering the pregnancy (Rs. 1000); second, after receiving at least one ANC (Rs. 2000), and finally, after childbirth (Rs. 2000).

Past studies have demonstrated the effectiveness of DBT in improving the use of antenatal check-ups, facility delivery, as also in reducing OOPE (Leone et al. 2013; Mohanty and Srivastava 2013), hence, a positive influence on health outcomes. There are, however, conflicting views on the association of DBT with maternal and neonatal health outcomes. Contrary to studies that have shown a positive impact of JSY on reducing neonatal deaths and improving newborn practices such as early initiation of breastfeeding and increased postnatal check-ups (Sen et al. 2020), other studies (Ng et al. 2014; Jackson et al. 2015) have observed no association of JSY with neonatal health outcomes. The economic impact of JSY is that families experience a marginal decline in delivery expenditure but spend more on medicines and transportation (Gopalan and Varatharajan 2012). In India—a country with a large population size, regional diversity in socioeconomic development and health systems—the coverage and effectiveness of such schemes (Thongkong et al. 2017) varies across the regions. Analysing the economic impact of DBT, the challenges in its implementation are extremely important in Bihar's socioeconomic milieu with existence of crippled health infrastructure.

In Bihar, the JSY scheme was launched as the Janani evam Bal Suraksha Yojana (JBSY) in 2006. Antenatal care use and institutional births have shown a tremendous increase post the implementation of JBSY. Seventy-nine per cent live births took place in a health facility as per NFHS-4 (2015–2016), compared to 39 per cent according to NFHS-3 (2005–2006), showing an increase of over 40 per cent in a decade. The survey data collected also supported the evidence and found a positive role of DBT in promoting the use of newborn health services.

> *The study showed that while neonatal deaths were fewer among the JBSY beneficiaries (19 per 1000 live births) than the non-beneficiaries (31 per live births) who had delivered in a public facility, the difference was not statistically significant. Therefore, a direct association of JBSY with neonatal mortality could not be established. However, in line with other studies, the significance of the programme in improving newborn care practices—such as early initiation of breast feeding, skin-to-skin care, postnatal check-ups, and birth weight monitoring—was observed. For instance, while 85 per cent mothers who had registered with JBSY and delivered in a public facility-initiated breast feeding, 82 per cent of the non-beneficiaries did so. Postnatal check-ups of newborns by community workers were also found to be higher among the JBSY beneficiaries (69 per cent) than the non-beneficiaries who had delivered in a public facility (45 per cent). The programme's effect on the birth weight of newborns delivered in a public facility could be observed as women enrolled in both PMMVY and JBSY reported lower birth weight of the baby (17 per 1000 live births) as*

compared to the non-beneficiaries (20 per 1000 live births). These evidences suggest that DBT played a critical role in newborn health in the study area.

Given the potential of the schemes to improve newborn care, there is an urgent need to examine the effectiveness of the schemes in reducing OOPE and the barriers to its implementation in the context of low socio-cultural and public health settings of Bihar. Evaluation of such schemes will provide directions to policy makers for introducing appropriate reforms in their implementation to bring about equity in healthcare. The respondents in the study site were hardly able to differentiate between JBSY and JSSK as most of them were well-informed about the cash benefits offered for institutional delivery under JBSY. Since PMMVY is a recently launched scheme, limited only to first birth, a major part of this chapter emphasises on JBSY. This chapter consists of three sections. The first section provides the status of and differences in the coverage of the schemes across the districts and socioeconomic groups. The second section explains the role of these schemes in reducing the burden of delivery expenditure. The third section identifies the impediments to the implementation and use of such schemes. Respondents' opinions/perceptions as to how such programmes can be better implemented are also discussed.

Coverage of DBT: Status and Differential

In 30 per cent of the villages surveyed, more than three-quarters of eligible households received DBT. A similar proportion of the villages (27.5 per cent), close to half or more of the households were covered by the JBSY scheme. Over three-fifths of the respondents (86 per cent) surveyed were aware of JBSY, while only 30 per cent had the knowledge of the PMMVY scheme. Nearly 10 per cent of the respondents were unaware of the financial interventions, and there were wide inter-district variations. Only 6.5 per cent women in Khagaria were unaware of JBSY, whereas the figure was three-fold higher in Rohtas and Kishanganj. More than three-fifths of the respondents were unaware of PMMVY irrespective of the districts surveyed. Lack of awareness was most observed in Khagaria (76.5 per cent), while it was comparatively low in Jehanabad (63 per cent) and Nalanda (64 per cent). This difference in knowledge of both the schemes could be attributed to the fact that PMMVY is a fairly recent programme, launched in 2017, just two years before the survey.

Of the total women who had delivered in a facility (whether a public facility or an accredited private facility), 56 per cent were registered with JBSY, 2.4 per cent were registered with PMMVY, and around 8 per cent were registered in both the schemes. Approximately 34 per cent respondents were not registered with any of the schemes. Of the women who had a public facility delivery, 9 per cent were not registered with any of these schemes. The proportion among them was the highest in Madhubani (13 per cent), followed by Muzaffarpur (10.4 per cent), while it was much lower in Rohtas (3.2 per cent). This raises the important question as to why a group of women who gave birth in a public facility did not opt for JBSY and why some women preferred home delivery despite having the knowledge of JBSY.

The analysis (Table 8.1) shows that among the registered beneficiaries, 71 per cent women benefitted from JBSY whereas only one-fifth had received the incentive under PMMVY that reflects the gap in service delivery. Around 63 per cent of respondents were beneficiaries of both the schemes. At least four among five deliveries in Kishanganj (83.5 per cent), Nalanda (83.8 per cent), and Jehanabad (80 per cent) were the JBSY

Table 8.1 Women registered and received benefit for facility delivery (in per cent)

District	*Registered with JBSY & received incentive for public facility delivery*	*Registered with JBSY & received incentive for private facility delivery*	*Registered with PMMVY & received incentive*	*Registered with both JBSY & PMMVY and received incentive*	*Received JBSY incentive within 30 days*
Jehanabad	80	17.3	32.9	68.8	64.5
Nalanda	83.8	17.3	7.7	72.6	57.2
Rohtas	55.4	0	37	38.2	23.9
Kishanganj	83.5	0	73.5	76.4	52.1
Madhubani	59.5	3.6	0	49.0	30.6
Muzaffarpur	59.6	13.4	0	50.2	34.9
Khagaria	73.2	25	0	70.6	22.4
West Champaran	60.7	0	20	54.0	21.2
Total	**71.3**	**7.4**	**19.5**	**62.7**	**39.2**
N	**1071**	**127**	**64**	**1426**	**882**

Source: Field data

beneficiaries while for other districts it was three out of five and the coverage was lower in Rohtas (55 per cent) followed by Madhubani (59.5 per cent), Muzaffarpur (60 per cent). A majority (76.4 per cent) of the beneficiaries in Kishanganj received benefits of DBT, while a low of 38.2 per cent did so in Rohtas.

Surprisingly, despite the introduction of the Public Finance Management System (PFMS), a digital platform for transferring cash benefits, most of the respondents reported delay in the receipt of payments. Almost 60 per cent beneficiaries reported receiving the payment after one month of delivery. Timely and early receipt of the incentive (within the first month of delivery) was reported the most in Jehanabad (64.5 per cent). In Khagaria, only 42.4 per cent of the beneficiaries received the money within 60 days. More than half of the respondents from Rohtas (55.5 per cent), Madhubani (52.2 per cent), and West Champaran (51.1 per cent) reported receiving money after 60 days. Around 29 per cent stated they did not receive the money, and 4.7 per cent reportedly received less than the full amount. This is evidence of the gaps that persist in the effective implementation of the schemes that affects use of MCH services. Perhaps, the financial illiteracy of the respondents also hinders their ability to stay updated about the amount received. Many of them depend on an ASHA facilitator to get the money. The non-availability of ASHA workers or their expectation of a commission for getting the benefit delivered to the beneficiaries' results in delays.

Socioeconomic Differentials in Utilisation of DBT

Ample evidences show that the structural and social determinants of health are the cause of inequities in the use of institutional care and access to financial benefits. The report of the 'Commission on Social Determinants of Health' provided a useful framework to address the inequities, and barriers to access, associated with maternal and newborn healthcare utilisation in the context of these schemes as they have a direct impact on health outcomes (WHO 2008). In low-income states of India, poor health indicators largely are the reflection of persistence of class and caste inequalities. Such inequalities compounded with inequities in other socioeconomic attributes impact access to various developmental opportunities, including DBT. In contrast to the established caste inequality in various health indicators, no significant caste differential was observed in the coverage of DBT in the study area (Table 8.2). More than three-fifths of the eligible

Table 8.2 Percentage of mothers registered for JBSY by socioeconomic differential

Socioeconomic profile	*Beneficiaries of DBT for facility delivery*	*P-value*
Educational status		**p<0.005**
Illiterate	67.5	
Primary	64.8	
Secondary	56.9	
Higher secondary & above	51.3	
Social group		**P<0.010**
SC/ST	62.8	
OBC	62.3	
General	64.4	
Expenditure class		**P<0.10**
Poorest	62.7	
Poor	64.9	
Middle	66.5	
Rich	59.0	
Richest	60.5	
Caste-class & education inequalities		
SC/ST*illiterate	61.0	
Non-SC/ST*illiterate	74.5	
SC/ST*poorest	57.5	
Non-SC/ST*poorest	70.1	
Poorest*illiterate	57.0	
Poorest*higher education	64.3	
Total	62.6	
N	**1426**	

Source: Field data

women, irrespective of their caste, received benefits under DBT. To be precise, the figures were 62.8 per cent (SC/ST), 62.3 per cent (OBC), and 64.4 per cent (General). Unlike with caste, JBSY coverage did differ in terms of education, with a higher number of the less-educated women (67 per cent) availing the benefits than those with higher secondary and above (51 per cent) levels of education. No significant economic differential was observed regarding the coverage of the scheme. Nevertheless, the disadvantages did manifest when considered in combination.

The intersection of the social determinants, such as caste-class, caste-education, or class-education, reveals the differential coverage of financial benefits and the least advantaged being more vulnerable in accessing the benefits. For instance, 61 per cent illiterate women from lower castes had access to DBT which increased to 75 per cent for illiterate women of general caste. Likewise, within the poor class, 57 per cent SC/ST women were covered by JBSY, whereas the figure increased to 70 per cent for non-SC/ST women. The intersection of social determinants—the societal causes intersecting with the system-level bottlenecks—contributes to inequalities in the uptake of maternal and child health, although the coverage extends to the lower economic strata (Mishra et al. 2021; Gupta et al. 2018). This again raises the important question as to why all the eligible women do not opt for institutional delivery to avail cash benefits under conditional cash transfer.

Out-of-Pocket Expenditure and Maternal and Newborn Care

High out-of-pocket expenditure on maternity and newborn services obstructs its utilisation, increases the maternal and neonatal health risk, and exacerbates the economic burden (Lim et al. 2010; Skordis-Worrall et al. 2011; Coffey 2014). Indian government has taken the responsibility of providing free maternal-newborn services, and it also provides financial help for reducing economic burden and preventing risk of maternal and newborn death. It has been brought to the fore that despite introduction of financial intervention and free services at delivery points, many families pay out of pocket (Leone et al. 2013; Jackson et al. 2015; Mukherjee and Singh 2018). The provision of services, including medicines, tests, and free food, encourages women to opt for institutional delivery and offset their expenses (Randive et al. 2013).

It is believed that since a decade and half over after the scheme introduced, perhaps these schemes, may help in reducing the economic burden of the poor in the state. *The significance of the programme in reducing the cost-of-service utilisation*[2] *was found positive in the study, suggesting that DBT plays an important role in reducing the economic burden of maternity and child care.* However, it does not cover the entire delivery expenditure. The mean OOPE for delivery in a public facility was estimated at Rs. 1509. The average expenditure on antenatal, delivery, and postnatal care

[2] A linear regression analysis was performed to see the association of out-of-pocket expenditure with JBSY after controlling for other socioeconomic factors such as education, caste, and place of delivery (results are not presented due to word constraints).

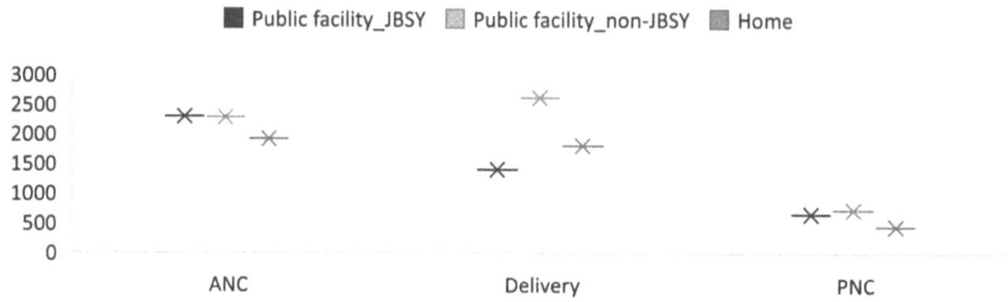

Fig. 8.1 Expenditure on ANC, delivery, and PNC by JBSY status. (Source: Field data)

for JBSY beneficiaries and non-beneficiaries who delivered in a public facility as well as those who delivered at home is presented in Fig. 8.1.

The total delivery expenditure in public facilities was around two times higher for the non-JBSY beneficiaries (Rs. 2619) than the JBSY beneficiaries (Rs. 1405). Even home delivery had a cost implication, with cost being higher than the cost incurred by the JBSY beneficiaries. It may be noted that in the case of home delivery, families paid a delivery fee or made in-kind payments (agricultural produce, new clothes, etc.) to the traditional birth attendants, called, in local terms, dais.

We estimated the monetary value of in-kind payments to get an estimate of the expenditure made on a delivery. No significant differences in the cost of ANC and PNC were observed by JBSY status.

One of the respondents who had a home delivery said:

> *We paid 30 kg anaj (grains) to the dai and also gave her the kind of new clothes she had asked for. We incurred more expenditure by having the delivery at home than we would have in a facility. Although a home delivery costs a lot more, we are not interested to go the hospital. Poor quality and high expenditure discourage us from going to the hospital.*

Another respondent, named Sangeeta Devi, from Jehanabad district stated:

> *We could not afford the cost of care at a hospital and, hence, decided to deliver the baby at home. But the dai charged us Rs. 1000 for conducting the delivery.*

In contrast to the perceptions that home delivery costs lower despite being covered by financial programmes, field information shows that the

JBSY recipients incurred lower expenditure than those who delivered at home or the non-beneficiaries who had a facility delivery. This underscores the importance of creating awareness regarding the access to financial schemes to reduce the burden of expenditure on maternal and newborn services. Like delivery expenditure, ANC and PNC expenditure were also relatively lower among the JBSY beneficiaries, although the differences were not striking. Respondents who had a home delivery made lower PNC expenditure than those who delivered at a facility irrespective of their access to JBSY. This indicates that the former had less exposure to PNC services perhaps due to a lack of awareness, or it could be that unaffordable cost of care reduced their propensity to visit a facility.

Moreover, being covered by JBSY reduces the burden of OOPE, but the family always pay out of pocket. Even though maternal health services are provided free of charge at public facilities, households in the study areas had to pay almost one-fifth of their budget share as OOPE for facility delivery. The previous chapter noted that the cost of medicines, followed by the cost of diagnosis, constitutes a major proportion of delivery cost irrespective of the care. The unavailability or less availability of medicines, and the practice adopted by doctors to involve more private players for profit, leaves the patients with no choice but to buy the prescribed medicines at a higher cost (Kotwani 2013), which leads to high OOPE. Informal payments made for or indirect expenditure incurred on delivery also cause higher OOPE.

While financial interventions play a positive role in reducing OOPE, the burden of spending is not equitable across the regions and economic classes. Most of the surveyed districts—like Madhubani (Rs. 2800), West Champaran (Rs. 2509), Muzaffarpur (Rs. 1738), and Rohtas (Rs. 1636)—recorded the highest expenditure on delivery. In contrast, the OOPE was the lowest in Khagaria (Rs. 632), followed by Nalanda (Rs. 900), Kishanganj (Rs. 990), and Jehanabad (Rs. 1178). The intra-regional differentials in health expenditure appeared due to the non-availability of facilities at the institutions that forced families to incur expenditure on their own.

The study data revealed a regressive pattern of the health spending where the lower class spent a larger share of their budget than the richest class. While OOPE was 1.12 times of the entire expenditure of the household for the poorest, the proportion of OOPE dropped to the extent of being half the total expenditure (0.53 times) among the richest. A relatively higher expenditure burden among the poor makes them vulnerable and reduces their likelihood of using MNCH services. The persistence of the economic inequality in delivery expenditure is corroborated by the results of many other studies (Skordis-Worrall et al. 2011). There was also a significant rural-urban differential in OOPE for delivery care, with urban households having incurred a higher expenditure (33 per cent of household budget) than their rural counterparts (24 per cent). In contrast, no expenditure inequality in OOPE was observed across the caste groups. Almost one-fourth of the household budget, irrespective of the caste, was spent as OOPE. The economic and geographical inequality in expenditure should, thus, be taken into consideration during the planning and implementation of similar health protection measures to ensure full coverage.

Barriers Affecting Utilisation of Programmes

This section documents the experiences of the women related to their reasons for not being enrolled and the challenges faced in accessing the benefit amount.

Lack of Awareness

Despite various community-level interventions—such as person-centred awareness generation by ASHA workers, putting up of hoardings, and execution of advertisements—lack of knowledge about the scheme surged as the most important reason for non-registration in the study. Approximately 14 per cent eligible beneficiaries were unaware of direct benefit transfers, with a disproportionate share of them being women of the low socioeconomic class. In line with the other studies (Kaushik et al. 2010), the present study found that low educational attainment among the poor and the marginalised was often the reason behind the low level of knowledge regarding the health needs of mother and newborn and hence, the low access to social assistance programmes. In addition, low level of communication on the part of the health workers acted as an impediment to the utilisation of the services by the less educated (Sharma et al. 2011). Nearly 6 per cent of the sample respondents stated that they were never informed about the programme by any health worker.

Insufficient Amount and High OOPE

Financial hardship is a major access barrier to healthcare services, which, in turn, has a significant influence on maternal and neonatal mortality. Among the potential beneficiaries around 16 per cent of those who had a facility delivery and 19 per cent of those who had delivered at home were not interested in JBSY due to low amount. Around 10 per cent who had availed stated the amount was not sufficient for meeting the expenses. The data also revealed that despite being covered by JBSY, families incurred a substantial OOPE on delivery. This signifies that even though DBT is meant to provide financial assistance to the poor, the stipulated amount is not sufficient to meet the cost of delivery care. Most of the women perceived the amount to be insufficient for reducing their cost of care and, therefore, preferred home care. Cost of care often comprises indirect expenses, such as those on hospital stay or food, or informal payments for services received. Many times, such informal payments are under reported. The disaggregated cost of delivery in a public facility, presented in Chap. 4, showed that almost 10 per cent of the total delivery expenditure was 'other expenditure'. It was observed from the field that such informal payments arose mainly due to the supply-side constraints. Families must make under-the-table payments for receiving quality services faster, and they are asked to contribute towards the cost of scarce supplies which are otherwise supposed to be provided for free. In addition, they are expected to offer gifts or tips to the health staff. These informal payments increase the cost of delivery in facilities and, therefore, the OOPE.

A JBSY beneficiary reported:

> *The amount given is helpful in reducing OOPE but not sufficient to reduce the burden of expenditure on delivery. It should be transferred before delivery so that we can utilise it to buy medicines or other items.* (Priyanaka Devi, Muzaffarpur)

Economic Inequality in OOPE

Shifting the burden of healthcare cost of newborns to the shoulders of poor who are already vulnerable has a significant impact on the use of services. Even though the financial interventions covered almost three-fourths of the respondents, women from the poorer strata faced more financial disadvantages as they had to bear relatively higher burden of

OOPE than the rich. The poor-rich equity ratio revealed that in public facilities, the delivery expenditure of the poorest was almost two times higher than that of the richest. For instance, OOPE on delivery constituted three-fourths of the household budget in the lower economic strata against 30 per cent among the richest. Such inequality in health expenditure not only discourages the poor from accessing institutional care, but also makes them impoverished and exacerbates the economic burden. To cope up with the delivery expenditure, 23 per cent households took loans, and around a fifth of them did so from a village moneylender at high rates of interest. Such compulsions push the households into the debt trap and, hence, lead to poverty.

Administrative Difficulties

Rigid administrative processes and fraudulent practices discourage women from availing the financial assistance. Despite opting for facility delivery, around 5 per cent of the women in the study reported that they and their families were not interested in the financial assistance mainly due to the administrative difficulties. Around 3 per cent of respondents had no bank account at the time of delivery and had no knowledge about how to open one. Financial illiteracy forced many poor women to depend on the community health worker for getting the incentive amount. A recurring complaint, however, was that the families were having to pay money to the health workers for assistance with receiving the money. Around 2.3 per cent said the commission asked for by the ASHA workers discouraged them from trying to get the benefit. This finding is corroborated by other studies that have found that community workers impose informal charges on women and their families (Coffey 2014). A study in the state of Jharkhand, carried out to find out the barriers to the coverage of JBSY, showed although some women were willing to opt for institutional delivery, several obstacles prevented the uptake of the JSY cash incentive and institutional delivery care such as poor infrastructure, poor quality of care, difficulties in accessing the cash incentive, and corruption in the disbursement of the incentives (Rai et al. 2011).

A woman from Madhubani had registered for PMMVY. Almost two years after the delivery, she claimed that the money had not been transferred to her, although her family paid Rs. 1000 to the ASHA worker to get the complete amount transferred to her.

Another respondent from Khagaria said that the ASHA *didi* did not communicate about the scheme properly. Also, the ASHA worker had taken Rs. 700 from her to get her the entitled amount of Rs. 1400.

One of the respondents described her experience:

> *I was interested to get the JBSY cash benefit. With the support of my family, I opened a bank account but did not fill out any form for JBSY. The ASHA worker was not supportive nor did she share her telephone number. My husband has to commute daily. There was no one else in the family to do the follow-up.* (Puja Devi, 20 years, Jehanabad)

A respondent who had a home delivery reported:

> *I was aware of the financial benefit for institutional delivery. But it is difficult to get the incentive amount as it needs paper work. I was not inclined to visit a facility for delivery for this reason.* (Manju Devi, 30 years, Nalanda)

Delay in Payment and Absence of Prepayment

The duration it takes for the incentive to reach a beneficiary is an indicator of how effective the implementation of the programme is. The delay in receiving the funds and the shortfall in the amount received compared to the entitlement may affect the correct utilisation of the programme. Only 39 per cent women in the study area received the incentive amount within 30 days. Among the registered beneficiaries of JBSY, more than one-fifth (22 per cent) reported administrative difficulty with receiving the benefit in a timely fashion. The State Health Society of Bihar, the implementing agency of the health programmes, found that in the initial years of the implementation of JBSY, there was a delay in processing the payment to the beneficiaries. The time it took ranged from two months to two years. To avoid those difficulties, the government is now investing into creating a digital infrastructure for the direct transfer of the benefits. The state has introduced the PFMS module to directly transfer the money to the bank account of the beneficiaries. However, there are challenges among the service recipients as well. Financial illiteracy of the beneficiaries, for instance, increases their dependence on community workers, which further lowers their ability even to know whether the transfer has taken place since the workers may not always be available.

In the survey, a majority (88 per cent) of the respondents reported that prepayment of the incentive would have benefitted them more as they could have utilised it from early in the pregnancy on things like nutritious food and medicines and would have been encouraged to access institutional care. The latest scheme, PMMVY, does have a prepayment component. The scheme, however, is limited only to the first child. Besides, in the Indian culture, women often move to their natal home during pregnancy. This too results in them remaining deprived of the PMMVY benefit as it is available to them only at the in-laws' place where they are registered with the scheme. A common barrier found in both the DBT schemes was that if the registration place varied from the birthplace, the eligible women registered with the schemes were not able to avail the benefits.

Discussion

The pro-poor programmes, implemented across the districts of Bihar, appear to be working as a catalyst in reducing the economic burden of facility delivery, improving newborn weight, and promoting care practices. Despite one and a half decades of implementation of JBSY in the state, challenges persist in terms of awareness, size, and equity aspects of the scheme. The findings show that the distribution of the gains from these interventions is insufficient and uneven across the economic classes, which reinforces vulnerability and widens inequality in the use of healthcare. In the absence of an adequate amount of financial protection, households rely exclusively on out-of-pocket expenditure, and the burden of OOPE is disproportionately high among the poor. The concentration of poor indicators adds to these vulnerabilities. Along with a rigid insistence on the bureaucratic processes, the obligation to make informal payments and the financial illiteracy among the beneficiaries discourage the poor from utilising such schemes.

While cash payments reduce the burden of OOPE, there is a need to rethink about the size of the amount and revisit the distribution mechanisms. The budgetary allocation to health, as a percentage of GDP, is 1.2 per cent in India, lower than even Bangladesh (1.3 per cent). This covers only one-fourth of the cost of healthcare services. As such, there is a large extent of distress financing despite JBSY (Mishra and Mohanty 2019), which serves only to discourage the utilisation of facility care. Increasing the amount of financial support, in the light of high OOPE among the poor as evident from the study, will be an encouraging step towards improved maternal and newborn health outcomes. Increasing the awareness about the processes of receiving entitlement will expand the coverage of the scheme. Tracking all the pregnancies through an online system and making payments irrespective of the birthplace will further help increase the coverage of the scheme. Timely and transparent disbursement of the cash benefit is important for reducing the complexities in the distribution of the benefits. A monitoring cell could be established at the block level to receive a monthly list of beneficiaries of the schemes. For ensuring a timely disbursement, the authorities in this cell could plan periodic monitoring visits to address the issues that delayed the process. The challenges of implementation drawn from the study have vital implications for future policy interventions and offer lessons to other countries with low rates of institutional delivery and poor reproductive health outcomes.

References

Borooah, V. (2010). Inequality in health outcomes in India: the role of caste and religion. In Thorat, S., Newman, K.S. (Eds.), *Blocked by caste—Economic discrimination in Modern India* (pp. 179–207). New Delhi: Oxford University Press.

Brearley L, Mohamed S, Eriyagama V, Elwalagedara R, Rannan-Eliya R P. *Impact of maternal and child health private expenditure on poverty and inequity* 2012. https://www.adb.org/sites/default/files/publication/30156/impact-maternal-child-health-private-expenditure.pdf

Coffey, D. (2014). Costs and consequences of a cash transfer for hospital births in a rural district of Uttar Pradesh, India. *Social Science & Medicine, 114*, 89–96.

Gaarder, M. M., Glassman, A., & Todd, J. E. (2010). Conditional cash transfers and health: unpacking the causal chain. *Journal of Development Effectiveness, 2*(1), 6–50.

Gopalan, S. S., & Varatharajan, D. (2012). *Addressing Maternal Healthcare through Demand Side Financial Incentives.*

Gupta, A., Fledderjohann, J., Reddy, H., Raman, V. R., Stuckler, D., & Vellakkal, S. (2018). Barriers and prospects of India's conditional cash transfer program to promote institutional delivery care: a qualitative analysis of the supply-side perspectives. *BMC Health Services Research, 18*(1), 1–12.

Huque, A. A. Z., Mavalankar, D., Kwast, B., & Hazra, M. (1996). *Evaluation report (Safe Motherhood Programme of India)*. Prepared for the Ministry of Health and Family Welfare of India. Washington, DC: MotherCare, John Snow Inc.

Hurst, T. E., Semrau, K., Gawande, A., & Hirschhorn, L. R. (2015). Demand-side interventions for maternal care: evidence of more use, not better outcomes. *BMC Pregnancy and Childbirth*, *15*(1), 1–14.
Jackson, P.T., Mazumdar, S., & Mills, A. (2015). Financial incentives in health: New evidence from India's Janani Suraksha Yojana. *Journal of Health Economics*, *43*, 154–169.
Kaushik, A., Mishra, C. P., Kesharwani, P., & Richa, H. M. (2010). Awareness about JSY among reproductive age women in a rural area of Varanasi. *Indian J Prev Soc Med*, *41*(3–4), 158–161.
Kotwani, A. (2013). Where are we now: assessing the price, availability and affordability of essential medicines in Delhi as India plans free medicine for all. *BMC Health Services Research*, *13*(1), 1–14.
Leone, T., James, K. S., & Padmadas, S. S. (2013). The burden of maternal health care expenditure in India: multilevel analysis of national data. *Maternal and Child Health Journal*, *17*(9), 1622–1630.
Lim, S. S., Dandona, L., Hoisington, J. A., James, S. L., Hogan, M. C., & Gakidou, E. (2010). India's Janani Suraksha Yojana, a conditional cash transfer programme to increase births in health facilities: an impact evaluation. *Lancet*. 5;375(9730):2009–23.
Mishra, P. S., Veerapandian, K., & Choudhary, P. K. (2021). Impact of socio-economic inequity in access to maternal health benefits in India: Evidence from Janani Suraksha Yojana using NFHS data. *Plos One*, *16*(3), e0247935.
Mishra, S., & Mohanty, S. K. (2019). Out-of-pocket expenditure and distress financing on institutional delivery in India. *International Journal for Equity in Health*, *18*(1), 1–15.
Mohanty, S. K., & Srivastava, A. (2013). Out-of-pocket expenditure on institutional delivery in India. *Health Policy and Planning*, *28*(3), 247–262.
Mukherjee, S., & Singh, A. (2018). Has the Janani Suraksha Yojana (a conditional maternity benefit transfer scheme) succeeded in reducing the economic burden of maternity in rural India? Evidence from the Varanasi district of Uttar Pradesh. *Journal of Public Health Research*, *7*(1).
Ng, M., Misra, A., Diwan, V., Agnani, M., Levin-Rector, A., & De Costa, A. (2014). An assessment of the impact of the JSY cash transfer program on maternal mortality reduction in Madhya Pradesh, India. *Global Health Action*, *7*(1), 24939.
Pathak, P. K., Singh, A., & Subramanian, S. V. (2010). Economic inequalities in maternal health care: prenatal care and skilled birth attendance in India, 1992–2006. *PloS One*, *5*(10), e13593.
Rai, S. K., Dasgupta, R., Das, M. K., Singh, S., Devi, R., & Arora, N. K. (2011). Determinants of utilization of services under MMJSSA scheme in Jharkhand 'Client Perspective': a qualitative study in a low performing state of India. *Indian Journal of Public Health*, *55*(4), 252.

Randive, B., Diwan, V., & De Costa, A. (2013). India's conditional cash transfer programme (the JSY) to promote institutional birth: is there an association between institutional birth proportion and maternal mortality?. *PloS One*, *8*(6), e67452.

Sen, S., Chatterjee, S., Khan, P. K., & Mohanty, S. K. (2020). Unintended effects of Janani Suraksha Yojana on maternal care in India. *SSM-Population Health*, *11*, 100619.

Sharma, P., Semwal, J., & Kishore, S. (2011). A comparative study of utilization of Janani Suraksha Yojana (maternity benefit scheme) in rural areas and urban slums. *Indian Journal of Community Health*, *23*(1), 11–14.

Skordis-Worrall, J., Pace, N., Bapat, U., Das, S., More, N. S., Joshi, W., … Osrin, D. (2011). Maternal and neonatal health expenditure in Mumbai slums (India): a cross sectional study. *BMC Public Health*, *11*(1), 1–12.

Thongkong, N., Van de Poel, E., Roy, S. S., Rath, S., & Houweling, T. A. (2017). How equitable is the uptake of conditional cash transfers for maternity care in India? Evidence from the Janani Suraksha Yojana scheme in Odisha and Jharkhand. *International Journal for Equity in Health*, *16*(1), 1–9.

WHO (2008) *Closing the gap in a generation: health equity through action on the social determinants of health: Commission on Social Determinants of Health final report*. Commission on Social Determinants of Health, & World Health Organization.

CHAPTER 9

Conclusion and Way Forward

Summary of Evidence

The mortality declines among newborns and their improved health has a great impact on the size of population and socioeconomic transformation of any country as a healthy start to life offers opportunities for human capital development and contributes to economic growth in the long run. Over the decades, improving MNCH outcomes in low-performing regions of the globe including India has been widely recognised. Great strides have been made in this direction as evidenced by plans and policy documents of the country. The sustained focus on MNCH care has resulted in a decline in maternal and child mortality, but the fundamental challenges to newborn survival remain the same, specifically in the resource-poor regions, albeit the intensity of the problem is declining. The estimation of Sharma and Gaur (2019) shows Uttar Pradesh, Madhya Pradesh, Bihar, and Rajasthan alone contribute to 55 per cent of total neonatal deaths in India and to 15 per cent of global neonatal deaths annually. Despite the significance of neonatal health, the linkages that determine newborn health and their survival chances have not been clearly established. To date, little research has been conducted to obtain a universally acceptable explanation of the impediments to newborn survival while considering the structural and societal complexities, where as the focus was more on bio-medical reasons. The present book attempted to fill the gap through a primary study of one of the resource-poor states of India—Bihar.

S. R. Mahapatro, *Towards Newborn Survival*,
https://doi.org/10.1007/978-981-19-3417-9_9

India is a country with diverse socio-cultural, economic, and political landscapes that each influences the performance of the health system differently. A crippled health system with increasing commodification of services—coupled with societal causes such as beliefs and norms, economic deprivation, and high population base—works together in perpetuating the mortality risk and poses challenges to bring down mortality rates among neonates. Uncovering the contextual barriers including health system bottlenecks, and their intricate relations, is thus critical to build a responsive health system and, therefore, improve health outcomes. At the beginning of this book, I answered questions regarding the societal and structural barriers, and their multifaceted interactions, that ail newborn survival in Bihar. In addition, I assessed the policy reforms in the health sector that impacted newborn health. The book offers insightful evidences on the linkages that impacted newborn health through a cross-sectional survey in eight sample districts of Bihar, selected based on their performance in terms of institutional births.

Neonates, as the most vulnerable group of children, entail special consideration from caregivers and also from the state. Neonatal mortality in Bihar fell 10 per cent between 2017 and 2018 after a gap as an outcome of various transformative measures. Its proportion of under-five deaths, however, remains stagnant and is higher than in many other states and higher than even the all-India average. To identify the causes underlying neonatal deaths, an overview of the social determinants of neonatal mortality, in low- versus better-performing states, has been presented in Chaps. 2 and 3. In doing so, the relative strength of the household, individual, and health system factors has been examined. Neonatal mortality is relatively high in the EAG states and is shaped by such attributes as wealth status, education, caste, and birth spacing. Prematurity/low birth weight was found to be the major cause of neonatal death and was linked to poverty, housing, environmental condition, and access to healthcare services.

Neonatal health disadvantages were experienced more among the poor and marginalised, as women belonging to such strata confront more access barriers. The intersection of the social dynamics meant that poor women, belonging to lower castes, were the least advantaged in terms of access to newborn health services. The question, thus, may be posed here as to why neonatal health disadvantages are experienced more by the poor and marginalised communities. In an industrialised society, higher socioeconomic status is linked to better health outcomes. It appears in a hierarchal society with resource crunch, living at the bottom level of the hierarchy leads to least access to resources. It is legitimate then to state that the pervasive social process determines healthcare access and the survival advantage often increases with the increase in the availability of better means. The causal association can be established as much through personal attributes of perception and attitude as through structural forces of poverty, inequality, health system functioning, and political leadership. These inequalities further might be the reflection of the failure of the health system to deliver health services to the poor. The interaction of these structural and economic forces creates and reproduces unequal health outcomes.

With a population of over 30 million living below the poverty line, mostly in rural areas (World Bank 2016), making MNCH services universal is challenging for Bihar. After almost 75 years of Independence, Bhore committees' recommendations were not appropriately implemented and reflected in the health system structure in terms of inequitable distribution and inefficient functioning. Given Bihar's status as an overpopulated state, the increasing demand for healthcare is exerting a bigger-than-ever pressure on PHCs, CHCs, and tertiary hospitals. Between 2009 and 2018, the population served per hospital and per bed almost doubled in the state. This indicates that merely increasing the capacity of the physical infrastructure, let alone is not sufficient, rather more resources should be infused for expanding human resources and improving the service delivery to meet the healthcare needs. The existing data collected on allocation of the healthcare resources demonstrates its uneven distribution across the districts and non-availability in many villages. The remoteness of a health centre from a village that ranges from 4.5 km to 10.2 km in the study discourages the poor households from going in for institutional care, unless had complications, as there are transportation costs and many times its simply unavailable. The significance of sick newborn care units to newborn survival highlights the need for providing specialised care at a low cost, ensuring early referral, and fostering community-facility linkage. Although SNCU centres have been set up across the state, their functionality and affordability require the attention of the state. Inadequate quality infrastructure, increasing cost of services, and skewed allocation are the major supply-side constraints of newborn services.

Insightful evidences from various studies reviewed in this book have documented that in a situation of high socioeconomic inequality, the pathways that influence newborn health negatively can be broken through the quality of services offered. Quality of care seems to be a supply-side barrier but the perception and trust that influence health-seeking behaviour are also influenced by QoC. Women can overcome other barriers if they perceive a facility as competent, effective, and safe (Bohren et al. 2014). Policy interventions of the state enormously have paved the way for progress in institutional deliveries; however, quality of care provided in the facility remained a neglected dimension and the evidences presented in the study reveal a scope for its improvement. Shorter length of stay, waiting time for registration, and the provider bias were other major difficulties found at facility. Despite the provision of free food & transportation under JSSK, the coverage was not universal. Only a quarter of women accessed ambulances, and a majority had to spend a huge amount of money to avail the services. Poor counselling at the time of discharge reduced the number of postnatal visits and affected the use of care practices. Despite higher cost, increasing utilisation of services from private facilities and dependency on informal service providers like quacks, locally known as jhola chaps, further reflect the poor service quality. Facility delivery alone, thus, cannot bring down deaths among neonates unless the QoC is prioritised.

Along with the inconsistent quality of services, misperceptions, traditional norms, and cultural practices shape the utilisation of newborn health services. TBAs are strongly preferred in many parts of rural Bihar for home delivery cases, while medical care is often considered as the last resort. Avoiding colostrum feeding, practising prelacteal feeding, bathing the baby as per traditional practices, putting kajal in the eyes, and following the traditional way of care for the umbilical cord (usually oil or ghee; most of the families applied a blue-coloured local medicine) were still prevalent in certain pockets of the study area. Confinement of women and children for a certain duration after delivery, as they are considered impure and polluted, reduced their postnatal visits. In spite of their biological advantage in longevity, female newborns experienced more early neonatal deaths than male newborns. This is a matter of concern for the state as it has one of the highest gender differences in mortality. Patriarchal norms and deep-rooted socio-cultural prejudices, such as son preference, result in a high level of gender discrimination against female newborns. The gender bias is also reflected in SNCU admissions apparently due to the prevailing gendered norms and the high treatment costs.

Home-based newborn care is one of the low-cost effective community interventions in resource-poor states that help change social norms and practices through knowledge and awareness, early detection of danger signs, and appropriate referral (Taleb et al. 2015). Its success has been noted in various South Asian countries like Bangladesh, Nepal, Pakistan, and India. One of the examples is cited by Bang et al. (1999), whereby three years of intervention in rural Gadchiroli of Maharashtra resulted in a 62 per cent reduction in neonatal mortality. Despite various efforts in the form of nukad natak, media coverage, and hoardings, the role played by community workers in spreading health knowledge and awareness was found to be a major demand-side barrier. Around 10 per cent respondents were not aware of antenatal visits, and more than one-third were not aware of PNC visits. The present study demonstrated that home visits of community workers (ASHA) fell far short of the protocol, with the average being one visit per household. Persistent socioeconomic inequality, low perceived need, and insufficient coverage of demand generation services thus paved the way for exploring the local and cultural factors affecting newborn survival.

The gradual commodification of healthcare makes utilisation of health services a costlier affair. Financial hardship and higher cost of services turned out to be the major barriers to newborn care and households' descent into poverty. The financial hurdles were particularly formidable for the marginalised in the study. CCT schemes introduced under NHM are expected to reduce the cost of delivery against the expectation; the latest NFHS-5 survey shows that OOPE increased from Rs. 1728 to Rs. 2848 between 2015 and 2020 in Bihar; the increasing trend was also observed in Andhra Pradesh and north-eastern states whereas the cost of delivery was declining in the western states. In the study, a major share of expenditure was seen to go to medicines, followed by diagnosis. For treatment of sick newborns at SNCUs, families face catastrophic expenditure, leading to distress financing such as borrowing and selling off assets, which push them into the debt trap and disincentive for admission.

The direct benefit transfer programmes have succeeded in overcoming the financial barriers, but to a limited extent. In the survey, DBT was found to cover only around 40 per cent of delivery expenditure and rest had to be made out-of-pocket. Pro-poor policies though designed to reduce financial barriers in delivery, the persistence of economic inequality in OOPE reflects the expenditure inequalities are pro-rich and healthcare costs is higher among the poor. This signifies the programmes are biased towards relatively better off and is the prerogative of the rich. Low purchasing power due to low income, compounded by high healthcare costs, has a huge implication for the newborn health in poor family. Ensuring equitable and universal coverage of maternal health services thus is a challenge for the poorest state Bihar. The study revealed that despite over one and a half decades of implementation, the direct benefit transfer was yet to reach almost 40 per cent of the respondents. Lack of awareness was the major reason for not registering, while almost 10 per cent of the potential beneficiaries were just not interested in the financial incentives. Studies have shown that covering treatment costs under DBT is usually insufficient for increasing the demand for treatment as the incentive remains unutilised by some women whose husbands do not want the stigma of being labelled as poor (Hunter and Murray 2017). In many instances, reaching the poor also remains a challenge due to local norms and beliefs that subvert institutional care for newborns. Along with a rigid insistence on the bureaucratic processes, financial illiteracy and informal payments discourage the poor from utilising such schemes.

The Way Forward

Regardless of how much improvement in MNCH care we have achieved, a holistic approach of health sector is required to meet the SDG targets of reducing neonatal mortality to 12 per 1000 live births by 2030. Given the findings, I want to put forth a few suggestions to resolve the challenges of newborn survival in the state.

Inclusion of Vulnerable and Underserved Groups

Despite its aim to achieve universal coverage, the health system of many countries follows the 'inverse equity hypothesis', whereby the benefits of a new intervention reach the better-off group first, while the poor are late recipients (Victora et al. 2000). Such approaches perpetuate inequalities in health outcomes. In Bihar the caste-class-based stratification is much prevalent and resources are limited; those at the bottom of hierarchy have least access to all resources including health. Although such challenges were recognised long ago at a global level and investments were made in this direction, inequalities in coverage and access till persist. Given the complexities of the social determinants, research and intervention should be designed within an intersectional framework for the universalisation of MNCH services. In the study, the preponderance of health disadvantages of newborns was evident among the marginalised. Alongside financial constraints, lack of awareness due to low levels of education and poorly perceived need for health resulted in the low utilisation of MNCH services. Future strategies, assuming further marginalisation, should be designed taking into consideration the barriers to delivering healthcare services to the underprivileged. The inclusion of the Mahadalits[1] into various maternal and newborn programmes is required for scaling up healthcare use among SCs/STs by bringing about behavioural change.

Enhancement of Coverage and Stringent Monitoring of CCT Schemes

Economically poor families burdened with higher relative disadvantages in OOPE for newborn health in the study indicate government schemes are not much help. Given these realities, the quantum of the incentive should be enhanced for the poor to lift them out of impoverishment. Together with this, delays in disbursement and the hidden cost of accessing the benefit, such as under-the-table or extra payments, constrain the beneficiaries from getting full advantage of a scheme. A monitoring cell may be established at the block level for ensuring a timely disbursement of the actual amount of the incentive through periodic monitoring visits. The extent of distress financing to meet delivery expenditure and, for SNCU treatment is substantial. Those families failed to meet the required expenses could not able to save the life of newborn. The state needs to introduce financial protection schemes for the sick newborns, specifically for the weaker section. There is a pressing need to formulate policy guidelines or to redesign the existing schemes to protect families from incurring substantial out-of-pocket expenditure on SNCU. Since medicines form a major component of expenditure, strengthening the drug procurement system will ease the availability of free medicines in all public health facilities and reduce the burden of OOPE on households.

Emphasis on Behavioural Change Interventions

Community health interventions influence positively newborn survival, however perform poorly in terms of coverage and knowledge of, and equity in, access to these interventions in the state. The health system of the states should, therefore, work in this direction to improve maternal and newborn health.

[1] Mahadalits are the poorest group of scheduled castes in Bihar. The term Mahadalit was introduced in Bihar by the Nitish government in 2007. The Bihar State Mahadalit Commission recommended the inclusion of 18 scheduled castes in this category. Mahadalits constitute an important group of voters in the state.

Family-Centric Approach

Behavioural change interventions for upscaling the utilisation of MNCH services should emphasise a family-centric rather than an individual-centric approach. Husband and in-laws are generally the immediate caregivers and decision-makers for the utilisation of MNCH services. The AWWs, PRIs, community leaders, and village health workers should involve and counsel the family members to make them realise the importance of timely ANC and PNC visits and of other scientific childcare practices under RMNCH+A, which will reduce the delay in seeking the services.

Women Empowerment and Intensified IEC Campaigns

Empowering women through education, livelihood opportunities, and media exposure enables them to make an informed choice about their own and their child's health. Mass media plays a decisive role in increasing awareness and, hence, results in empowerment. The study found that majority of the women from the low socioeconomic class were not aware of any SMS facility providing information on maternal and child care. This shows that *Kilkari*, the mobile health education service (m-Health programme) designed to help new and expecting mothers with healthcare choices, is not successful. Efforts thus should be directed at disseminating simple-yet-effective and easy-to-understand IEC material in the local languages through popular print and digital media to ensure a wider coverage of the illiterate population. Besides, creating a mass awareness campaign in the Jan-Andolan mode is required to increase the demand for MNCH services.

Strengthened Community Engagement

Collective involvement and participation of communities is known to increase newborn survival in many parts of the globe, including India. In Bolivia, a programme named 'Warmi' resulted in a decline in neonatal mortality with a participatory approach (Howard-Grabman 2002). The success of such an approach is also evident in eastern India, where states like Odisha and Jharkhand launched a programme named Ekjut trial (2005–2008) that resulted in a 45 per cent reduction in NMR (Tripathy et al. 2010). In Bihar too, there exist initiatives with a participatory approach, but women are neither aware of them nor actively participate in the community meetings. Involvement and counselling of PRI members and SHG workers in VHSND sessions and setting up of health camps will lead to sensitisation of the community towards the special maternal and child needs. The PRIs and other stakeholders of the society should be a part of the counselling sessions and be convinced to motivate the masses to discard the deep-rooted culture of son preference.

Community-led transport mechanisms can improve access to emergency obstetric care like in Ghana and Tanzania. Community prepayment schemes can be a support to poor households in reducing their expenditure burden. An emergency fund can be created in every village for the use of ambulance services, especially for pregnant women located in remote villages and those belonging to the weaker sections. Funds from the Rogi Kalyan Samiti can be utilised for the same. The state should replicate the successful models of other states and countries for newborn survival.

Transformative Measures for Eliminating Gender Disparities

Like the PCPNDT Act that was implemented to reduce female foeticide, strict laws should be enforced to check female infanticide (covering the neonatal period and infancy). Similar to the education promotion and empowerment schemes like Beti Bachao Beti Padhao, Mukhyamantri Kanya Utthan Yojana, plans/schemes may be introduced for the free vaccination and medical treatment of the girl child up to age five to reduce gender inequality in newborn and infant care. This gender disparity can further be eliminated by IEC campaigns and women empowerment. Instead of viewing a girl child as a burden, the community should be shown to accept and rejoice in the birth of a female just like that of a male. ASHA should broach gender disparity issues in Gram Sabha meetings and encourage the community to eliminate gender disparity in the utilisation of healthcare services.

Promotion of Home-Based Newborn Care Practices

Community health workers (CHW) play a key role in counselling pregnant women on healthy lifestyles, birth planning, complication readiness, ANC, skilled care at birth, and postnatal practices. This helps create links between the community and the healthcare system. The coverage of newborns through such programmes is helping reduce neonatal mortality in

Bihar. However, the coverage falls well below the protocol as, on an average, an ASHA worker makes only 1.3 visits per household during the postnatal period. These shreds of evidence suggest that the standard protocol of home visits by link workers should be rigorously implemented. An online system can be created to track HBNC visits received by a newborn. The system would yield case-wise data for the beneficiaries of the HBNC programme and bring transparency to it. Overburdening of the ASHA workers, due to workforce shortage and payment of low compensation to them, affects the effective implementation of the intervention. A simple form of appreciation for the best-performing ASHAs and an increase in the compensation paid to them will boost their morale and ensure that they work more enthusiastically for reaching the goals.

Strengthening of the Health System

Scaling Up of Infrastructure

Despite long period after Bhore committees' recommendation, till now non-availability and skewed allocation of healthcare resources is a central challenge to meeting the health goals in Bihar. Financial incentives alone cannot generate demand for MNCH services unless there is an upsurge in physical and human resources in the health sector. For instance, as per Rural Health Statistics (2019–20), the shortage of ASHA workers was around 15 per cent in the state. Though they are the backbone of the health system, they are underpaid and overburdened, which hampers the effective implementation of the programmes. In the public facilities, long waiting times, improper staff behaviour, lack of ambulance, and shorter length of stay due to inadequate infrastructure were the major negative experiences recounted by the respondents in the study. The capacity of the health system should be strengthened through investment in physical and human resources. Emphasis should be placed on improving the networking linkages between healthcare providers at each level (primary, secondary, and tertiary) so that they can attend to the complications of women and sick newborns immediately. A complete referral system must be in place that includes transportation, experts, medicines, and equipment at the desired referral centre.

Increase in Health Budget

Health is a public good in India, and a major stakeholder of public health facilities are the poor. Nevertheless, given the high cost and the poor quality of care at facilities, the tendency to use public facility declines even among the deprived section of the community. The poor quality of services, which is linked to the low public health expenditure, forces a segment of the lower economic strata to utilise private facilities in the state. NFHS results show that an increasing proportion of the rural poor are visiting private facilities for delivery (from 10 per cent in 2005–2006 to 13 per cent in 2015–2016). The field data also supports this with the evidence that around 17 per cent of poor households chose private facilities as the place of delivery. Compounding the problem is the high cost of seeking SNCU treatment of newborns, which leads to the impoverishment of families and reinforces their vulnerability and makes a substantial out-of-pocket expenditure.

The structural bottlenecks of the health system that make the health service delivery inefficient can be overcome by increasing the budgetary allocation, which is, of course, very low in Bihar. The public expenditure on health for the entire period under NDA rule in Bihar has remained, on average, less than 4 per cent of the total state expenditure. With the shift to a market economy in pursuance of structural adjustment programmes, private healthcare was promoted more pronouncedly with the reduction in public health expenditure. Currently, the state has upsurged the health budget due to the emergence of the COVID-19 pandemic with medical spending crowding out other sectors' spending to meet the crisis. The increased spending if continued in a sustained manner perhaps benefited the poor and the marginalised in accessing health services including MNCH care. The experiences of the public healthcare system—as it exists in a country like Cuba, which is, itself, a cash-starved nation—can be immensely rewarding in providing credible support to develop a feasible healthcare model for rural Bihar.

Tracking and Screening of Every Pregnancy

ANC is the first point of contact between mothers and the health system and offers an opportunity to develop a birth emergency preparedness plan whereas the state is one of the lowest in full ANC. Besides, the coverage of other integrated services, such as HIV tests, hepatitis, and diabetes, was significantly low in the study. Early detection of high-risk pregnancy through proper tracing and screening is possible by increasing the coverage of ANC and conducting all the tests in a timely manner. Reducing the barriers through increase in awareness, provision of free diagnosis, and expansion of transportation services will increase ANC coverage, reduce dropouts, and strengthen the ANC intervention.

Standardisation of Training and Mentoring of Providers

One of the main obstacles to newborn survival is the prevalence of home deliveries that are conducted largely by TBAs where the government initiatives are undermined. Many countries—including Burkina Faso, Cambodia, Indonesia, Morocco, and Sri Lanka—have significantly reduced maternal and newborn deaths by training and deploying midwives. Providing training to the local traditional birth attendants/dais about early newborn care will help improve home-based newborn care. The study clearly shows that mothers in contact with ASHA/ANM/ health personnel have better outcomes in overcoming the traditional barriers and providing their newborn with more essential care both pre- and post-delivery. Monitoring of activities of the health workers should be carried out periodically to keep them updated on the latest innovations related to essential and immediate newborn care practices.

Disease-Specific Interventions in the National Health Programmes

A detailed death audit is required at the village level to understand the cause of death of newborns who die at home. The survey data showed that 30 per cent of deaths were due to unknown reasons since those deaths were not registered nor medically certified. The audit will help gain clarity on the burden of specific illnesses/diseases of the newborn. Prematurity/ LBW was the major cause of death in the study and was linked to poverty of, and poor nutrition and anaemia in, mothers. Interventions for promoting family planning, encouraging healthy dietary habits, and reducing child marriage reduction are needed. Cause-specific interventions may be integrated into the national health programmes to make quality care available for all.

Bihar has made notable progress in public health indicators; yet the health sector needs major reforms on many fronts. A sustained focus on child health programmes has resulted in a decline in infant and under-five mortality, but improvement in newborn survival is modest. In a vast country like India, with a considerable demographic and socioeconomic diversity, one-size-fits-all approach may not be able to address the barriers to newborn health, whereas state-specific measures are highly desirable. Like that of many low-resource regions with fiscal limitations, the health system of Bihar confronts a continued pressure on the infrastructure, which is marked by poor quality, deficit budget, and unequal distribution of services and poor governance. In conjunction with this, the prevailing socioeconomic system and institutions perpetuate inequalities in health outcomes. Theoretically, in a scenario with high-income inequality, the diffusion of innovations in the health sector is slower for the poor than the rich. Till date the issue of neonatal mortality is always linked to biomedical reasons, not put in a larger link to societal factors such as poverty, livelihood, and inequality. Further, during the pandemic life of majorities is affected by falling employment opportunities, and reduced income has amplified the newborn care challenges. To lower NMR, a holistic approach—considering economic, socio-cultural and health system barriers—is needed.

In the current scenario, the overall social milieu and political environment of the state play an important role in setting the priorities and directions for improving health system. Government's investment mostly focuses on construction of building, while pay limited attention to their functionality that affects quality-of-service delivery. Further, the political parties often announce many schemes around elections with a lack of understanding about their effective implementation within limited resources. Instead, policy agenda for improving MNCH indicators should be more realistic. Policymakers of the state should, thus, restructure the health system, and the state should allocate resources for the universalisation of RMNCH services in future. Moreover, unless the political economy of the health system of the state is addressed systematically, it may be difficult to improve health outcomes, including neonatal health.

References

Bang, A. T., Bang, R. A., Baitule, S. B., Reddy, M. H., & Deshmukh, M. D. (1999). Effect of home-based neonatal care and management of sepsis on neonatal mortality: field trial in rural India. *The Lancet*, *354*(9194), 1955–1961.

Bohren, M. A., Hunter, E. C., Munthe-Kaas, H. M., Souza, J. P., Vogel, J. P., & Gülmezoglu, A. M. (2014). Facilitators and barriers to facility-based delivery in low-and middle-income countries: a qualitative evidence synthesis. *Reproductive Health, 11*(1), 1–17.

Howard-Grabman, L. (2002). Community organization and perinatal outcomes in Bolivia: the WARMI project. *Journal of Perinatology, 22*: S20–4.

Hunter, B. M., & Murray, S. F. (2017). Demand-side financing for maternal and newborn health: what do we know about factors that affect implementation of cash transfers and voucher programmes?. *BMC Pregnancy and Childbirth, 17*(1), 1–28.

Rural Health Statistics. (2019–20). Published by Ministry of Health and Family Welfare, Statistics Division, Government of India.

Sharma, A. K., & Gaur, A. (2019). Profile of neonatal mortality in special newborn care unit of tertiary care hospital, *International Journal of Contemporary Pediatrics, 6*(6), 2319–2325.

Taleb, F., Perkins, J., Ali, N. A., Capello, C., Ali, M., Santarelli, C., & Hoque, D. M. E. (2015). Transforming maternal and newborn health social norms and practices to increase utilization of health services in rural Bangladesh: a qualitative review. *BMC Pregnancy and Childbirth, 15*(1), 1–11.

Tripathy, P., Nair, N., Barnett, S., Mahapatra, R., Borghi, J., Rath, S., ..., Costello, A. (2010). Effect of a participatory intervention with women's groups on birth outcomes and maternal depression in Jharkhand and Orissa, India: a cluster-randomised controlled trial. *The Lancet, 375*(9721), 1182–1192.

Victora, C. G., Vaughan, J. P., Barros, F. C., Silva, A. C., & Tomasi, E. (2000). Explaining trends in inequities: evidence from Brazilian child health studies. *The Lancet, 356*(9235), 1093–1098.

World Bank. (2016). 'Bihar: Poverty, Growth and Inequality'. World Bank. http://documents.worldbank.org/curated/en/781181467989480762/pdf/105842-BRI-P157572PUBLIC-Bihar-Proverty.pdf

Index[1]

[1] Note: Page numbers followed by 'n' refer to notes.

S. R. Mahapatro, *Towards Newborn Survival*,
https://doi.org/10.1007/978-981-19-3417-9

FSC
www.fsc.org
MIX
Papier | Fördert gute Waldnutzung
FSC® C083411

Kolibri 360 GmbH
Ferdinand-Jühlke-Straße 7
99095 Erfurt, Deutschland
produktsicherheit@kolibri360.de